Theoretical Perspectives on Language Deficits

Issues in the Biology of Language and Cognition
John C. Marshall, editor

Theoretical Perspectives on
Language Deficits

Yosef Grodzinsky

A Bradford Book
The MIT Press
Cambridge, Massachusetts
London, England

This book was set in Times by The MIT Press, using computer disks provided by the author, and was printed and bound in the United States of America

Library of Congress Cataloging-in-Publication Data

Grodzinsky, Yosef.
  Theoretical perspectives on language deficits / Yosef Grodzinsky.
    p. cm.
  Includes bibliographical references.
  ISBN 0-262-071123-1
  1. Agrammatism. 2. Psycholinguistics. 3. Neurolinguistics.
I. Title.
RC425.5.G76 1989
616.85'52—dc20   89-39398
                                                              CIP

To my parents

Contents

Foreword by John C. Marshall

The reception of modern syntactic theory by the (other) psychological sciences constitutes a fascinating, albeit bizarre, chapter in the history of intellectual endeavor. Noam Chomsky's early work (Chomsky 1957, 1965) had an immediate and electrifying impact upon studies of language perception and production (Miller, Galanter, and Pribram 1960; Morton 1964; Wales and Marshall 1966). Investigations of first language acquisition (Bellugi and Brown 1964) received a new lease on life; studies of aphasia (Goodglass and Hunt 1958; Marshall and Newcombe 1966; Whitaker 1969; Traill 1970) likewise took notice that a new and relevant theory was being formulated.

In retrospect, some of this work did perhaps "apply" the model a little naively. The problems of the "derivational theory of complexity" are real, although often exaggerated (see Berwick and Weinberg 1983); grammars written for children's speech looked more like utterance-cataloguing devices (Harris 1957) than the product of general laws; the competence-performance dichotomy was persistently misinterpreted despite the efforts of Chomsky (1965) and Fodor and Garrett (1966) to outline a straightforward distinction between what is computed in language use and how it is computed.

Nonetheless, the combination of a successful theory (Lees 1957) and a devastating attack upon the pretentions of Skinnerian behaviorism (Chomsky 1959) launched the cognitive revolution. Yet by the mid-1970s the interest of psychologists in transformational grammar had dwindled. All manner of strange devices—pragmatics, speech acts, schemas, perceptual strategies—were deployed to avoid confronting the plain fact that the core of a language is its syntax. Linguists were thus later compelled to reiterate the obvious. Gleitman (1981) quotes from a letter to TV Guide:

How Ann Salisbury can claim that Pat Lauder's anger at not receiving her fair share of acclaim for Mork and Mindy's success derives from a fragile ego escapes me.

And she glosses the remark with the observation that "this writer knows that the first 27 words determine absolutely that the 28th ends with an *s*.." Try accounting for that without invoking the notion of syntactic structure!

In part, the retrograde step of attempting to explain language acquisition and use without the constructs of formal grammar was taken because the theory of syntax was undergoing rapid change throughout the 1970s. Standard Theory was followed by Extended and Revised Extended Standard Theory, by Trace Theory, and the first major attempts to achieve explanatory adequacy by imposing severe constraints upon transformations and other rules of grammar (Chomsky 1977). But psychologists responded to the excitement of the times by withdrawing into their shells. A popular text (Clark and Clark 1977) acknowledged the existence of syntax but interpreted experiments on language performance in terms of constructs that could be found in any traditional grammar from Apollonius Dyscolus to Jespersen (1924). Johnson-Laird (1977) then took the ultimate step of arguing that psycholinguistics could be undertaken without linguistics!

Such responses to advance are, to put it mildly, peculiar. Yet Chomsky (1982) detected much the same reaction within linguistics itself, asserting that the discipline lacks "a widespread understanding of what is taken for granted in the natural sciences, namely that theory is going to change if it's to stay healthy. Many linguists feel that if a theory is proposed, tested and abandoned, or modified that shows that there is something wrong with the field." This odd attitude was then compounded when psychologists convinced themselves that their methods were intrinsically better than those employed by linguists.

The old issue of the "psychological reality of linguistic constructs" reemerged with full force. Householder (1966) had claimed that "A linguist who could not devise a better grammar than is present in any speaker's brain ought to try another trade." Psychologists now argued that even linguists who would not be more profitably employed in some other field were unfit to produce "psychologically real" grammars: to evaluate "internal" evidence about the structure of sentences and constraints upon grammatical form is merely to play with formalisms; to collect "external" evidence about "responses" to utterances is the touchstone of the "real." For psychologists of this ilk, Chomsky (1978) noted:

Certain types of evidence are held to relate to psychological reality, specifically, evidence deriving from studies of reaction time, recognition, recall, etc. Other kinds of evidence are held to be of an entirely different nature, specifically, evidence deriving from informant judgments as to what sentences mean, whether they are well formed, and so on. Theoretical explanations advanced to explain evidence of the latter sort, it is commonly argued, have no claim to psychological reality, no matter how far-reaching, extensive or persuasive the explanations may be and no matter how firmly founded the observations offered as evidence.

From that point of view, *only* evidence from molecular genetics is relevant to the claim that constraints on Universal Grammar are innate; *only* evidence from physiology or "behavior" (as construed by a methodological behaviorist) is relevant to a claim about the mental representation of *wh*-clauses. The whole sorry story is well known and I shall not elaborate upon it here, except to remark

that such an interpretation of "psychological reality" would, in ea
destroyed the development of perceptual theory across the board
psychophysics to the Gestalt laws of form. Let us turn instead to
and more cheerful, matters.

Explanation in the psychobiology of language must perforce s   ......ow
path between innate determinants of ontogenetic language growth and the
environmental truism that English is not Japanese. Thus, Universal Grammar
must account for the diverse forms of attested grammars within constraints that
allow them to develop on the basis of limited environmental triggering. Government Binding Theory took the first tentative steps toward meeting these demands
(Chomsky 1981). "We hope," Chomsky (1982) writes, "that it will ultimately be
possible to derive complex properties of particular natural languages, and even
to determine the full core grammar of a language with all of its empirical
consequences, by setting the parameters of general linguistic theory (universal
grammar, UG) in one of the permissible ways."

Recent studies have explored the nature of parameter setting in some detail
(Hyams 1986; Roeper and Williams 1987), with the consequences that developmental psycholinguistics is now a far more sophisticated enterprise than it was
in the 1960s. "Language acquisition is once again becoming an exciting growth
area, with the prospect of real convergence between linguistic theory and other
branches of psychology" (Smith 1988). Can we make the same claim for studies
of language impairment?

In the first modern text psycholinguistics, Fodor, Bever, and Garrett (1974)
made sweeping criticisms of all aphasiological investigations:

It is the sad truth that remarkably little has been learned about the psychology of language
processes in normals from over a hundred years of aphasia study, and that nothing at all
has been learned about possible neurological realizations of language from the psycholinguistic advances which this book will survey.

Even at the time, these reflections were overly gloomy (Marshall 1977), and it
quickly became apparent that linguists were taking an interest in the diverse
forms of acquired aphasia. Kean (1977) drew attention to the fact that traditional
characterizations of "agrammatism" in Broca's aphasia are ad hoc and fail to
make reference to any well-defined level of linguistic representation. Her own
suggestion was that the tendency to omit closed-class morphemes (bound and
free) could be uniformly interpreted as the simplification of sentences into
minimal strings of "phonological words."

Kean's theoretical proposal that agrammatism could be characterized at a level
of representation on the boundary between syntactic and phonological structures
did not go unchallenged. Alternative (or perhaps complementary) accounts of
the phenomenon began to proliferate. Lapointe (1983) argued that agrammatism
was better interpreted in terms of a unified theory of morphology; Caplan
(1983a) outlined a lexical hypothesis; and many students provided evidence for

"word-order" deficits in agrammatism that seemed to imply a syntactic locus for the problem (Saffran, Schwartz, and Marin 1980; Caplan 1983b).

This ferment is reflected in a volume edited by Kean (1985). The book draws attention to a variety of competing accounts of agrammatism, raises important issues about the nonhomogeneity of patients so classified, and discusses the relationships between impairment (and preservation) of linguistic form in language production, comprehension, and grammatical judgment. Subsequently, the controversy has continued unabated (Stemberger 1985; Lapointe 1985; Caplan 1986; Badecker and Caramazza 1986; Lukatela, Crain, and Shankweiler 1988; Nespoulous et al. 1988), drawing upon an ever-increasing body of rich empirical evidence (McCarthy and Warrington 1985; Ostrin and Schwartz 1986; Tyler and Cobb 1987; Berndt et al. 1988; Miceli et al. 1989). This debate, much of it now taking place within the overall framework of Government-Binding Theory (Grodzinsky 1986; Sproat 1986; Jarema, Kadzielawa, and Waite 1987; Caplan and Hildebrandt 1988; Martin et al. 1989) is exceptionally healthy. True, no consensus has yet been reached about the "correct" characterization of any aphasic impairment. But the issues are now debated with a rigor that was unimaginable even ten years ago. And it is no longer even halfway plausible to imagine that "external" evidence from aphasiology should be excluded from the data base of grammatical theory (Fromkin 1988), the inverse error to the psychologists' dismissal of "internal" evidence.

It is against this background, then, that Yosef Grodzinsky's *Theoretical Perspectives on Language Deficits* should be welcomed. Like so much of the recent neurolinguistic literature, the book focuses on "agrammatism in Broca's aphasia," but its scope is far wider. Grodzinsky carves out a position for the centrality of explicit linguistic theory in any study of language impairment. And he is unstinting in his criticism of other approaches (information-processing psychology, connectionism, and gross lesion-function correlationism) that have not paid sufficient attention to the nature of the representations made available by the language faculty.

This leads to a lucid overview of Government-Binding Theory, which is then applied in detail to the formal description of agrammatic speech production and comprehension. Grodzinsky's own position is sharply compared and contrasted with a wide range of earlier characterizations. Consider, for example, the status assigned to passives in different syntactic theories. In Lexical-Functional Grammar, both adjectival passives (*John was interested in Mary*) and verbal passives (*John was kicked by Mary*) are derived by lexical rules; but in Government-Binding Theory only the former is lexical, whereas verbal passives are transformationally derived. Grodzinsky shows that agrammatic aphasics can cope with adjectival passives almost as well as with actives, yet comprehension of verbal passives is at chance. Such patterning thus meets Grodzinsky's "Breakdown-compatibility constraint" if we assume that the relevant grammatical generalizations are as hypothesized in Government-Binding Theory rather than in Lexical-

Functional Grammar. Throughout, the chief concern is that, in addition to meeting the obvious constraints of observational and descriptive adequacy, accounts of "aphasic" language should be well grounded in general linguistic theory; aphasiology is not some specialized domain, divorced from the rules, representations, and processing mechanisms postulated to underlie normal performance.

This position leads naturally to a discussion of the "modularity thesis" as applied to neuropsychological data. The discovery of "how the brain cuts the syntactic pie" (to employ Grodzinsky's formulation) will place "severe restrictions on the class of biologically feasible grammars." And finally, Grodzinsky reopens the debate on the inverse relationship between language growth and language dissolution. The so-called regression hypothesis has not attracted a large number of supporters in recent years, but this reformulation of the issue from the standpoint of parallels between parameter acquisition and parameter loss will undoubtedly reinvigorate the argument.

Many of Grodzinsky's specific proposals will, I trust, prove highly controversial; as he himself writes, the thesis of *Theoretical Perspectives on Language Deficits* is not intended to be "the final word." Vendryes (1925) once wrote that "it is wrong to think of the brain as if it were built on the plan of a grammar, cut into sections for the different parts of speech." Perhaps . . . but maybe not so wrong as to think that the human brain is not built on the plan of a grammar.

References

Badecker, W., and A. Caramazza (1986). A final brief in the case against agrammatism: The role of theory in the selection of data. *Cognition* 24, 277–282.

Bellugi, U., and R. Brown, eds. (1964). *The acquisition of language.* Lafayette, IN: Child Development Publications.

Berndt, R. S., A. Salasoo, C. C. Mitchum, and S. E. Blumstein (1988). The role of intonation cues in aphasic patients' performance of the grammaticality judgment task. *Brain and Language* 34, 65–97.

Berwick, R. C., and A. S. Weinberg (1983). The role of grammars in models of language use. *Cognition* 13, 1–61.

Caplan, D. (1983a). Syntactic competence in agrammatism: A lexical hypothesis. In M. Studdert-Kennedy, ed., *The neurobiology of language.* Cambridge, MA: MIT Press.

Caplan, D. (1983b). A note on the "word order problem" in agrammatism. *Brain and Language* 20, 155–165.

Caplan, D. (1986). In defence of agrammatism. Cognition 24, 263–276.

Caplan, D., and N. Hildebrandt (1988). *Disorders of syntactic comprehension.* Cambridge, MA: MIT Press.

Chomsky, N. (1957). *Syntactic structures.* The Hague: Mouton.

Chomsky, N. (1959). Review of *Verbal behavior* by B. F. Skinner. *Language* 35, 26–58.

Chomsky, N. (1965). *Aspects of the theory of syntax.* Cambridge, MA: MIT Press.

Chomsky, N. (1977). *Essays on form and interpretation*. Amsterdam: North Holland.

Chomsky, N. (1978). On the biological basis of language capacities. In G. A. Miller and E. Lenneberg, eds., *Psychology and biology of language and thought*. New York: Academic Press.

Chomsky, N. (1981). *Lectures on government and binding*. Dordrecht: Foris.

Chomsky, N. (1982). *The Generative Enterprise*. Dordrecht: Foris.

Clark, H. H., and E. V. Clark (1977). *Psychology and language*. New York: Harcourt Brace Jovanovich.

Fodor, J. A., T. G. Bever, M. F. Garrett (1974). *The psychology of language*. New York: McGraw-Hill.

Fodor, J. A., and M. F. Garrett (1966). Some reflections on competence and performance. In J. Lyons and R. J. Wales, eds., *Psycholinguistics papers*. Edinburgh: Edinburgh University Press.

Fromkin, V. (1988). How relevant is "external evidence" for a theory of grammar? In C. Duncan-Rose and T. Vennemann, eds., *On language*. London: Routledge.

Gleitman, L. R. (1981). Maturational determinants of language growth. *Cognition* 10, 103–114.

Goodglass, H., and J. Hunt (1958). Grammatical complexity and aphasic speech. *Word* 14, 197–207.

Grodzinsky, Y. (1986). Language deficits and the theory of syntax. *Brain and Language* 27, 135–159.

Harris, Z. S. (1957). Co-occurrence and transformation in linguistic structure. *Language* 33. 283–340.

Householder, F. W. (1966). Phonological theory: A brief comment. *Journal of Linguistics* 2, 99–100.

Hyams, N. M. (1986). *Language acquisition and the theory of parameters*. Dordrecht: Reidel.

Jarema, G., D. Kadzielawa, and J. Waite (1987). On comprehension of active/passive sentences and language processing in a Polish agrammatic aphasic. *Brain and Language* 32, 215– 232.

Jespersen, O. (1924). *The philosophy of grammar*. London: Allen and Unwin.

Johnson-Laird, P. (1977). Psycholinguistics without linguistics. In N. S. Sutherland, ed., *Tutorial essays in psychology*, vol. 2. Hillsdale, NJ: L. Erlbaum Associates.

Kean, M. -L. (1977). The linguistic interpretation of aphasia syndromes: Agrammatism in Broca's aphasia, an example. *Cognition* 5, 9–46.

Kean, M. -L., ed. (1985). *Agrammatism*. New York: Academic Press.

Lapointe, S. G. (1983). Some issues in the linguistic description of agrammatism. *Cognition* 14, 1–39.

Lapointe, S. G. (1985). A theory of verb form use in the speech of agrammatic aphasics. *Brain and Language* 24, 100–155.

Lees, R. B. (1957). Review of *Syntactic structures* by N. Chomsky. *Language* 33, 375–407.

Lukatela, K., S. Crain, and D. Shankweiler (1988). Sensitivity to inflectional morphology in agrammatism: Investigation of a highly inflected language. *Brain and Language* 33, 1–15.

McCarthy, R., and E. K. Warrington (1985). "Category specificity" in an agrammatic patient: The relative impairment of verb retrieval and comprehension. *Neuropsychologia* 23, 709–727.

Marshall, J. C. (1977). Disorders in the expression of language. In J. Morton and J. C. Marshall, eds., *Psycholinguistics series*, vol. 1. London: Elek.

Marshall, J. C., and F. Newcombe (1966). Syntactic and semantic errors in paralexia. *Neuropsychologia* 4, 169–176.

Martin, R. C., Wetzel, W. F., Blossom-Stach, C., and Feher, E., 1989. Syntactic Loss Versus Processing Deficit: An Assessment of Two Theories of Agrammatism and Syntactic Comprehension Deficits. *Cognition* 32, 157–191.

Miceli, G., M. C. Silveri, C. Romani, and A. Caramazza (1989). Variation in the pattern of omissions and substitutions of grammatical morphemes in the spontaneous speech of so-called agrammatic patients. *Brain and Language* 36, 447–492.

Miller, G. A., E. Galanter, and K. Pribram (1960). *Plans and structure of behavior*. New York: Holt.

Morton, J. (1964). A model for continuous language behaviour. *Language and Speech* 7, 40–70.

Nespoulous, J. -L., M. Dordain, C. Perron, B. Ska, D. Bub, D. Caplan, J. Mehler, and A. R. Lecours (1988). Agrammatism in sentence production without comprehension deficits: Reduced availability of syntactic structures and/or of grammatical morphemes? A case study. *Brain and Language* 33, 273–295.

Ostrin, R. K., and M. F. Schwartz (1986). Reconstructing from a degraded trace: A study of sentence repetition in agrammatism. *Brain and Language* 28, 328–345.

Roeper, T., and E. Williams, eds. (1987). *Parameter setting*. Dordrecht: Reidel.

Saffran, E. M., M. F. Schwartz, and O. Marin (1980). The word order problem in agrammatism: II. Production. *Brain and Language* 10, 263–280.

Smith, A. (1988). Language acquisition: Learnability, maturation, and the fixing of parameters. *Cognitive Neuropsychology* 5, 235–265.

Sproat, R. (1986). Competence, performance and agrammatism: A reply to Grodzinsky. *Brain and Language* 27, 160–167.

Stemberger, J. P. (1985). Bound morpheme loss errors in normal and agrammatic speech: One mechanism or two? *Brain and Language* 25, 246–256.

Traill, A. (1970). Transformational grammar and the case of a Ndebele speaking aphasic. *Journal of the South African Logopedic Society* 17, 48–66.

Tyler, L. K., and H. Cobb (1987). Processing bound morphemes in context: The case of an aphasic patient. *Language and Cognitive Processes* 2, 245–262.

Vendryes, J. (1925). *Language: A linguistic introduction to history*. London: Routledge and Kegan Paul.

Wales, R. J., and J. C. Marshall (1966). The organization of linguistic performance. In J. Lyons and R. J. Wales, eds., *Psycholinguistics papers*. Edinburgh: Edinburgh University Press.

Whitaker, H. A. (1969). On the representation of language in the human brain. Doctoral dissertation, UCLA, Los Angeles, CA.

Acknowledgments

I would like to express my deepest gratitude to the individuals and institutions whose help, encouragement, and support were indispensable during the preparation of this book. The linguists among them kept me honest on linguistic issues; the psychologists, on matters psychological. Hagit Borer, Hiram Brownell, and Edgar Zurif read parts of the manuscript and commented on it extensively. Conversations I had with Noam Chomsky, Stephen Crain, Lyn Frazier, Howard Gardner, Merrill Garrett, Kyle Johnson, Beth Levin, David Pesetsky, Steve Pinker, Tanya Reinhart, Luigi Rizzi, Doug Saddy, Barry Schein, Peggy Speas, Max Taube, and Ken Wexler forced me to think harder and benefited me with many ideas. Special thanks go to Lyn Frazier and Virginia Valian, who gave the book a fair, constructive, and thorough review, and to Anne Mark who did an extraordinary job editing the manuscript. Some of the material presented here comes from articles coauthored with Yu-Chin Chien, David Finkelstein, Susan Marakovitz, Alexander Marek, Janet Nicol, Amy Pierce, Ken Wexler, and Edgar Zurif. I thank them all for their cooperation.

I had the good fortune to present some of the topics discussed in this book at various conferences: The Academy of Aphasia meetings in Los Angeles and Nashville, BABBLE in Niagara Falls, GLOW in Brussels, The North Eastern Linguistic Society at MIT, and the Cognitive Conference in Tel Aviv. Other matters were taken up in colloquia at the Aphasia Research Center, Boston University School of Medicine, the University of Connecticut, Johns Hopkins University, University of California at Irvine, UCLA, MIT, Carnegie-Mellon University, City University of New York, Bar Ilan University, and Haifa University. Comments from audiences at these meetings had a clear impact on the quality of the final product. Students in my linguistics and psychology classes at Tel Aviv University pressed hard and forced me to clarify matters for them, and for myself.

Without the help of friends this book would never have seen the light of day. Neora Berger rescued me from every computer trouble, Faye Bittker, Daniel Roth, and Efrat Tourjman came through with technical help at the last minute, and the others kept reminding me that the things of real importance are actually elsewhere.

Finally, I would like to acknowledge the support of National Institutes of Health (NINCDS) through grants NS 06209 and 11408 to the Aphasia Research Center, Boston University School of Medicine, and grant NS 21806 to Brandeis University, the Charles Smith Family Foundation at the Israel Institute for Psychobiology, the Bat Sheva de Rothschild Fund for Science and Technology, and the Sloan Foundation's particular program in Cognitive Science at the Center for Cognitive Science at MIT. The Center was exceptionally hospitable to me, for which I am most grateful.

Theoretical Perspectives on Language Deficits

Chapter 1

Introduction

1.1 Beginning

This book is about a set of natural phenomena, their proper treatment and theoretical relevance. It discusses neurological deficits that impair some mental faculties, deals with issues concerning their adequate description, and proposes ways they can inform various cognitive theories. In general, the discussion centers around the role neuropsychological evidence should play in theory construction in cognitive science. Conceptual as well as methodological problems arise when neurological findings and theoretical issues are confronted. As the story unfolds, it reveals a view of the proper form of argumentation, from cognitive deficits to cognitive theories.

This is the kind of phenomenon the book handles: A normal, fully functioning adult, whose cognitive capacities are mature (and not yet deteriorated from old age or senility), becomes brain damaged as a result of some physical event. This individual now exhibits abnormal behavior in one or more cognitive domains. The extent and type of the abnormality are determined, in part, by the size of the lesion, its locus, and so forth. They may range from total loss of function—blindness, muteness, deafness, quadriplegia—to partial loss. It is the latter boundary that is of interest to cognitive scientists, for it usually offers them a window through which they can peer into a part of the cognitive machine and get a glimpse of some of the processes that underlie our mental life.

If brain-damaged patients are willing to let us examine their behavior and test their partially impaired abilities, we are likely to observe phenomena that not only are inherently fascinating but also may be instrumental in theory construction, as they may reveal patterns of aberrant behavior that are theoretically relevant.

Identifying such interesting patterns, though, needs more than just a good eye. For such a pattern to be theoretically relevant, certain prerequisites must be met:

there must be a *theoretical question*, a *descriptive framework*, and a *method*. All three are defined, of course, relative to a theory. Little can be gained through mere "objective" observation of patients, or from presenting them with arbitrarily selected tasks designed to measure their behavior. Interest in neuropsychological disturbances lies in their *selectivity*, which is always described in theoretical vocabulary. Theories are just like beholders: they see beauty in different things. Impairment of one type may be relevant to one theory yet completely orthogonal to issues defined by another.

Instead of asking, then, whether a particular type of patient can or cannot perform some task (a common practice in the field), we must look at a set of behaviors, describe them in some theoretical vocabulary, and generalize to a theory. And if the latter is detailed and tightly constrained, we might find our generalizations significant. Assuming our theory to be about some mental faculty, it should make predictions about the kinds of selective impairment to that faculty that are possible and those that are not. Our theoretical knowledge teaches us, for example, that engines cannot be hemiplegic. That is, an engine cannot break in such a way that only its right side works. Yet we know that people can. This is because our theory of mechanics (and knowledge of the structure of engines) is different from our theory of the structure of the human central nervous system. Likewise, cognitive theories differ in their predictions about patterns of selective impairment to mental faculties.

This offers an excellent testing ground for theories. For inside every cognitive model, there is a tacit theory of cognitive impairment: the internal structure of the model—the arrangement of natural classes formed in it—determines which deficits are possible and which are not. In order to actually test theories, we play a game, whose rules are really simple: Take a syndrome that offers prima facie evidence for being relevant, describe the impairment pattern using theoretical vocabulary, derive predictions to test the description, so that it is refined and made precise, and then test the theory to see whether it in fact predicts the previously described impairment pattern. This is just what I do in this book, focusing on one aphasic syndrome: agrammatism in Broca's aphasia.

I first consider general conceptual issues pertaining to the theoretical relevance of neurological phenomena, language deficits in particular. Then I offer a formal description of agrammatism and discuss its implications for theories of language structure, processing, and acquisition. So, although the range of applications I discuss is relatively narrow, the argument I develop is actually quite general and can be applied to any cognitive domain, to the extent that relevant patterns of selectivity subsequent to brain damage are found in that domain.[1]

1.1.1 Differing Points of View

My argument will have other implications as well. One of them might seem depressing to some neuropsychologists, but to me it is actually good news: specifically, the claim that neuropsychology and neuropsychological phenomena do not constitute a separate domain of inquiry but instead represent a methodology that cuts across cognitive domains. I would also like to argue that the evidence provided by research into cognitive pathologies is doomed to be no more than auxiliary to theory construction. On this view, neuropsychological research takes advantage of naturally caused situations that allow certain experimental procedures and observations, which are otherwise impossible. If neuropsychology is about psychological disturbances that accompany physical damage to parts of the nervous system, and if domains of inquiry are defined by theories, then neuropsychology cannot constitute an independent domain.

Traditional positions on the role of behavioral pathologies are quite different and in fact are diametrically opposed to this view. Acquired cognitive deficits, particularly linguistic ones, have historically intrigued two groups of students. As acquired deficits, they have been considered topics of medical inquiry. That is, since the phenomena in question are all pathologies caused by some physical damage to the central nervous system, all of them were first observed by physicians and taken to be in the domain of clinical neurological research. Psychologists entered the scene later. Their interest in impaired psychological functions brought them in, and naturally they have tended to focus not on anatomical and physiological aspects of the phenomena but on their relation to the psychology of the organism.

Roughly corresponding to these two groups of researchers, two views on the role of behavioral aberration in theory construction can be identified. The first, held mainly by those who follow the well-known Wernicke-Lichtheim model for language (see Geschwind's celebrated 1965 article; Benson 1979; and other works cited below), takes the domain of empirical inquiry—aphasic, agnosic, or apraxic syndromes—as the main explicandum of the psychological (and anatomical) theory. Theories about the language faculty are inspired by observing the aphasias, alexias, and agraphias; motor theories are designed to account for the apraxias; and so on. No confirmation of these models is sought through observation of normal behavior, and little attention, if any, is paid to the relationship between normal and impaired cognitive functions. Neuropsychology, to these students of brain-behavior relationship, is at the theoretical centerstage.

The second position regarding the theoretical status of neuropsychological evidence argues that since the goal of psychological theory is to construct models that explain behavior, then by plain analogy, the goal of neuropsychology is to explain pathological behavioral patterns that arise following damage to some part of the central nervous system. Thus, the literature is replete with models that purport to "explain a syndrome."[2] It seems to me, however, that talking about neuropsychological theory, under these assumptions, is like talking about a special theory of computation for broken computers. Attempts to explain abnormal behavior arising from cerebral lesion by an independent neuropsychological theory are thus tantamount to efforts to explain how broken cars work. Such endeavors are probably possible (and potentially interesting to some), but their scientific relevance is far from clear. We are committed to accounting for the performance of brain-damaged patients, but we must do so by using modified models of the normal function. Otherwise, we will end up with one theory for normal functioning and another, unrelated theory for deficits. Neuropsychological phenomena should be described by independently motivated theories, their role in theory construction being a constraining one.

My view is diametrically opposed to both approaches. It judges the interest that a neurological phenomenon holds by its relevance to independently motivated theories of the normal cognitive function, thus allocating a much more modest role to neuropsychology. It sees neuropsychological evidence not as central to cognitive theories but as potentially accessory. Moreover, it does not take for granted the relevance of cognitive deficits to theories of human cognition. In this respect, it places the burden of argument on the neuropsychologist: a cognitive theory is committed to account for neuropsychological disturbances only if patterns of selective impairment can be demonstrated that are in the domain of the theory.

This work differs from others in another way as well. Each line of inquiry is naturally embedded in a general conceptual framework, and as these change, new issues in the study of cognitive pathologies emerge. The topics discussed in the field range from classical questions of cerebral localization of psychological functions, to the proper division between various cognitive domains, to yet newer questions regarding the identification of cognitive deficits with disruptions to specific loci in models of the functional architecture of the mind. Therefore, just as investigations of the nineteenth-century students—Broca, Wernicke, Lichtheim, and their colleagues—touched on questions formulated in the traditional theoretical vocabulary of neurology, so this work deals with questions that were formulated in relation to current approaches to cognition. It seeks neuropsychological evidence that can be brought to bear on matters that are discussed in the cognitive sciences. It differs from other studies in that it views cognitive deficits through the spectacles of the cognitive science of the 1980s. The difference will become apparent as we go along.

1.1.2   What Evidence Is Relevant?

Once a new theoretical perspective is introduced in the study of cognition, a question immediately arises for the neuropsychologist: Is there any relevant neuropsychological evidence, and if there is, how is it identified? Clearly, that acquired cognitive deficits would be an indispensable source of evidence for theory construction in cognitive science is not a logical necessity. One could imagine a whole host of possible cerebral pathologies (for instance, the case of total loss of function mentioned earlier) that are orthogonal to any psychological question. On the one hand, then, not every pathology of the brain is interesting to the cognitive scientist. On the other, there need not be a relevant deficit for every theoretical question. In fact, most theoretical debates are conducted without any neuropsychological evidence at all. The reasons are quite obvious: what determines the ultimate nature of a deficit is the physical properties of the damage to the central nervous system (size and location), and the locus of any such injury is determined by factors that are, in all likelihood, arbitrary from the point of view of cognition. That is, the distribution of blood vessels in the brain and the patterns of their injury (by clogging and rupture—the most common etiologies among those lending themselves to psychological investigation) do not appear to have anything to do with our mental structure. Thus, the claim that neuropsychological phenomena are relevant to cognitive theories is far from trivial.

The immediate result of this situation is that the theoretical relevance of pathological phenomena must be established on a case-by-case basis. One could, in fact, imagine a situation where no pathology would be relevant to cognitive theories. Despite this grim possibility, the evidence currently available at least from aphasic syndromes is quite suggestive. As we will see, the data show surprisingly fine distinctive patterns, which are relevant to central issues in theories of language structure, acquisition, and processing, in that they are a source of powerful constraints on these theories.

Some might think that if my argument is correct, then neuropsychological research should be dispensed with altogether. However, I believe this is exactly the opposite of what should be concluded. If my arguments are valid, then the role of the study of neuropsychological phenomena is made clear, and this study is seen as an important source of constraints to be imposed on cognitive theories. Instead of resulting in its dissociation from other branches of cognitive science, the view of neuropsychological research as an operation in the service of broad theoretical issues is beneficial to all parties concerned.

Now that we have looked at some general issues, it is time to focus on language. In the remainder of this introduction I will consider two topics. First

I will review some fundamental changes that the language sciences have undergone, and their consequences for the work of the practicing neuropsychologist. Then I will discuss conceptual problems that the description of cognitive deficits raises for the theoretician.

1.2   Conceptual Changes in the Approach to Language and Their Consequences

Until about thirty years ago it was generally believed in psychology that linguistic behavior was simply a result of conditioning and that one could not speak of knowledge that such behavior presupposes. The scene in American psychology was dominated by behaviorists, who were, as Jerry Fodor once dubbed them, "closet ontological purists," refusing to admit mental constructs into their models. Consider the way psycholinguists function in such a setting. Minds cannot exist under behaviorism. Therefore, grammatical rules do not exist, because they need minds in which to be represented. Moreover, behaviorist psycholinguists cannot assume that language comprehension and production consist, among other things, of rule-based analysis, because such assumptions are simply inconceivable within this conceptual framework. Language is thus seen as a set of almost trivial *practical abilities*. Behaviorists can speak of people uttering, understanding, repeating, naming, reading, and writing, but they are barred from analyzing the details of the process of comprehension, which cannot be based on represented knowledge. It is easy to see why linguists and psycholinguists had virtually nothing in common in the heyday of behaviorism. Linguistics was about discovery procedures for the structure of languages, whether English, Arabic, or Swahili, regardless of who spoke them, whether humans, apes, or Martians. By comparison, psycholinguistics was dedicated to exploring language behavior, which inheres in the linguistic activities that humans exhibit, and to describing the differences and similarities among these activities. The disconnection was perfect: linguists were interested in languages, not humans; psycholinguists were interested in human behavior, not in language.[3]

Given this background, it is not surprising that nineteenth-century accounts of language deficits, focusing on linguistic activities and ignoring grammatical notions, were very appealing to neuropsychologists at the time. These accounts saw language as a collection of activities and therefore characterized the various language deficits by patterns of impairment: one syndrome was described as a language production impairment, another as a comprehension impairment, and so on. Again, no explicit reference was made to linguistic elements or rules.[4] The neuropsychologists of language found these descriptions of selective language impairment patterns attractive and sensible, since they were fully consistent with the behaviorist conception of language.

Chomsky's attack on behaviorism in psychology and linguistics led to a major conceptual shift in the study of language and to the subsequent rise of mentalistic theories of language structure, acquisition, and processing (for a review, see Chomsky 1986a, chap. 2). Using the Cartesian "poverty of the stimulus" argument, he pointed out that humans have the ability to produce and understand sentences they have never heard and that such phenomena cannot be explained by the behaviorist stimulus-response paradigm. He (and others) also showed that the grammatical structure of human language is too complex to be learned just by analogy, as some (for example, Quine) had proposed. He concluded that human linguistic behavior is best explained by mentally represented knowledge and that in order to explain language acquisition, one must assume the existence of innate knowledge, which he called *Universal Grammar*. Thus, instead of being a collection of "practical abilities," whose acquisition is rather trivial and occurs via the application of simple analogical rules, "knowledge of language" is knowledge of a set of highly abstract principles that is claimed to uniquely explain the human ability to deal with the intricacies of language. Chomsky (1965) defines the subject matter of linguistic theory under this view as follows:

The problem for the linguist, as well as for the child learning the language, is to determine from the data of performance the underlying system of rules that has been mastered by the speaker-hearer and that he puts to use in actual performance. Hence, in the technical sense, linguistic theory is mentalistic, since it is concerned with discovering a mental reality underlying actual behavior. Observed use of language or hypothesized dispositions to respond, habits, and so on, may provide evidence as to the nature of this mental reality, but surely cannot constitute the actual subject matter of linguistics, if this is to be a serious discipline. (p. 4)

From the psychological angle, Fodor and Garrett (1966) made a very similar point:

There is no reason at all to suppose that, because the evidence for psychological claims is (often) the occurrence of one or another bit of behaviour produced by some organism, psychology is therefore primarily in the business of arriving at generalizations about behaviour. On the contrary, psychology is primarily concerned with understanding the nature and capacities of the mechanisms that underlie behaviour and which presumably cause it. (p. 136)

The outcome of this change is that explanations of observed behavior now focus on mental states and processes rather than on links between observed external events themselves. This shift has immediate consequences for the study of language behavior. If in the old framework predicates describing linguistic behavior and ability are monadic—that is, "John speaks, listens, reads, or writes"—then so is the predicate in "John knows L." Under this conception, it makes sense to talk about John's linguistic activities without referring to properties of L, because knowledge of language is an unanalyzed concept. However, if it is agreed (under the Chomskyan view) that grammar is mentally represented, then it makes no sense to speak of the linguistic activity without referring to the knowledge that is necessary for the activities to be practiced. It thus follows that the predicate in "John knows L" is a dyadic (two-place) predicate; that is, the theory describing John's linguistic abilities assumes knowledge of a set of grammatical principles. Therefore, talking about linguistic activities cannot be done without referring to grammar. The description of language behavior is now of the form "John produces, comprehends, etc., sentences of L."

If neuropsychologists accept Chomsky's arguments, then their focus and argumentation must change. The characterization of neuropsychological disturbances as impairment to activities is obviously inadequate. If before one could describe an aphasic syndrome as a disorder of speech production, for instance, now such a description will not suffice. Aphasic syndromes must be described in terms of "impairment to the ability to comprehend L (or parts thereof), sparing of the ability to produce L (or parts thereof)," and so on. This realization not only leads to the immediate rejection of the classical syndrome descriptions but also opens a new set of questions, both theoretical and empirical.

1.3   Three Approaches to Cognitive Deficits

1.3.1   Connectionism

Consider, first of all, the theories proposed by the *connectionist* school to account for human linguistic abilities (Wernicke 1874; Lichtheim 1885; Geschwind 1965, 1979; and many others). These theories see the mental structures responsible for observed cognitive skills as a collection of independent processes that underlie a variety of activities. These processes are believed to be well localized in cortex. In fact, the task of the theoretician, as seen by this school, is to identify the precise locus of cognitive processes in the brain. A cognitive theory, then, is a set of statements that associates activities (and hence processes underlying them) with specific brain sites and structures, and language is a collection of single processes, each underlying an activity (speech production, comprehension, reading, repetition, and so on). These activities are the basic theoretical terms, and they are specified as such without justification.

Acceptance of the linguistic activities as the building blocks of the theory is far from innocuous. In particular, it completely dismisses the possibility that the signal that these activities transmit (the linguistic signal) has any interesting properties of its own. In other words, according to these theories, language is use. Therefore, the neuropsychological evidence they seek consists entirely of dissociations among the various linguistic activities that humans engage in: loss of the ability to read without loss of the ability to write, and vice versa, points to distinct mental structures for the two; a consistent lack of distinction between abilities suggests a single structure responsible for the two. Finally, each activity is identified (roughly) with a brain area.

Figure 1.1 illustrates Geschwind's version of connectionism, superimposed on the left cerebral hemisphere. Four important observations concerning these theories: (1) Their methodology motivates theoretical distinctions through observations of patterns of selective impairment. (2) The set of data that is brought to bear on these theories is highly selective. Only specific kinds of data are relevant. In particular, finer-grained distinctions—impairment patterns whose description refers to aspects of the linguistic signal itself (that is, to grammatical elements)—are completely irrelevant, since this class of theories is incapable of handling them. Indeed, connectionist theories have never made reference to grammatical rules or elements. (3) Knowledge (linguistic or otherwise) plays no role in the explanation. (4) The conjectured activities are directly associated with cerebral regions.

Some of these observations constitute the very basis for rejecting connectionism as a theory of brain-behavior relations. Even though the internal logic of connectionist models looks appealing, there are several reasons to reject them. First, the formulation of the theory is based on some intuitive, undifferentiated notions of what underlies our linguistic abilities. Witness the words of Norman Geschwind, the main proponent of this approach in our time: "The notion that we need to know what language is before we ask where it is has little to justify it"

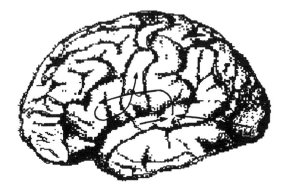

Figure 1.1

(Geschwind 1983, 62). The choice of theoretical terms—the units of analysis the theory offers—is unmotivated.

Second, this approach denies the relevance of grammatical variables taken from theories of linguistic representation to both the description of language deficits and theory construction. In light of the previous discussion, we can say that such a theory views knowledge of language as a one-place relation. Thus, it conflicts sharply with current views on language. Linguistic utterances are structured according to grammatical principles that are recruited to the service of each activity. To take some well-worn examples, (1) and (2) differ greatly in meaning, although they differ minimally in form.

(1) John is too stubborn to talk.
(2) John is too stubborn to talk to.

There is nothing in the particular channel of linguistic communication that determines the semantic contrast between these two sentences. Rather, the comprehension and production of such well-formed utterances must be guided by a particular kind of knowledge. Linguistic knowledge, then, is intimately tied to linguistic activities. Incorporating linguistic variables into the characterization of language deficits not only makes them more precise; it also shows that connectionism is false. Aphasia does not necessarily destroy the ability to communicate linguistically through a given channel, as connectionism would predict. Rather, it results in partial impairments to speech production, selective disruptions to the comprehension abilities, and so on. In fact, it will become apparent that the partition between the impaired and preserved abilities that underlie aphasic performance (at least in some central cases that are better understood than others) must refer to grammar. This observation clearly argues against connectionism, which claims that the linguistic activities are unanalyzed and therefore predicts that if an activity is disrupted, the disruption should be total. This prediction is false: Broca's aphasics, suffering from the paradigmatic "speech production" disorder, are not mute. Rather, the utterances they produce are aberrant from a *grammatical* point of view.

Finally, this approach assumes a trivial, one-to-one relation to hold between the functional characterization of behavior and the neural tissue supporting the mechanisms that underlie behavior. It does this by claiming that functions simply "live" in designated cerebral regions. It seems to me, however, that one must be much more cautious in relating different levels of analysis one encounters in modeling brain and behavior. Although there is something dramatic in the statement that the ability to create sentences lives in a particular cerebral center, there is no reason to suppose that the mapping between linguistic activities and brain areas is one-to-one. The state of the evidence at this point—the complicated patterns of selectivity observed after brain damage—does not warrant such a conclusion. More important, though, mere localization does not amount to explaining behavior. It is like stating that a particular racing car won the Indy 500 because its engine was in the front, without specifying any of its properties—a statement that may be true, but has a very limited explanatory force, if any.

As a theory of mental structure, then, connectionism should be abandoned.

1.3.2 Information Processing

Next let us examine a class of models known as *information-processing* models (Caramazza and McCloskey 1985; Coltheart, Patterson, and Marshall 1980; Morton 1982; Patterson 1981; and many others). These theories are about the functional architecture of the mind. Their goal is to provide causal explanations of behavior in terms of the flow of information from the distal stimulus into the mind, and from there up to the generated behavior. The statements they provide are thus in the form of flowcharts, where lines and arrows stand for the paths through which information flows and boxes stand for processes that manipulate information. The source of data for these models is both normal and pathological behavior.

In normal individuals, evidence usually comes from reaction-time studies, error analyses, and so on. With respect to neuropsychological evidence, the methodology is basically identical to that of the connectionist models: distinctions drawn by the brain motivate processing distinctions (see Caramazza 1984). Yet the information-processing approach aims at analyses of behavior that are finer-grained than those of connectionism. In the domain of language, for instance, the goal is to analyze each activity into its component parts (from a functional point of view). Such models also acknowledge that the analysis of the language comprehension and production systems must involve grammatical variables. In addition, they make no commitment to anatomical localizationist claims. Rather, they are restricted to functional analyses of behavior. Since the data base for these models is both normal and pathological behavior, their empirical coverage and motivation are substantially broader than those of connectionism.

To see what an information-processing theory looks like, let us briefly review proposals to account for acquired dyslexia.

Acquired dyslexia is a reading disorder that is observed following brain damage. Similar to other cognitive deficits, it manifests itself as a selective disorder, thus providing the psychologist an opportunity to tease apart knowledge sources and processes involved in the complex activity of reading. As Patterson (1981, 158) clearly articulates it, "The aim of the cognitive psycholo-

to assign interpretations to input sentences. This is one of the most basic tenets of any computational system. Yet the information-processing models, which are claimed to provide "computationally explicit" models of cognitive processes, fail to meet this fundamental requirement. Missing from virtually all of these models is a schema that details the ways processes make contact with the knowledge base. Not only do they refer only vaguely to the knowledge base, as noted earlier; indeed, the part it should play in cognitive functioning is not clear. Again, the distinction Chomsky makes between monadic and dyadic theories of language is appropriate here. Denying the relevance of grammatical knowledge amounts to treating linguistic knowledge as an unanalyzed term and hence characterizes information-processing models as "monadic"theories.

As an example, consider once again the "grapheme-to-phoneme conversion" process of Patterson's (1981) proposal. In order to provide an explicit model, one must provide a set of such conversion rules and an algorithm that implements them. There are two ways of doing this. First, one could propose a conversion rule system for a particular language. Such a proposal would be rather narrow in scope. More abstractly, one could propose a universal characterization of grapheme-to-phoneme conversion rules. To do that, one would need to carry out a thorough investigation into the writing systems of the world and their relation to phonology.

John Marshall has made such an attempt. Realizing that "a theory of orthography should characterize both the universal constraints and allowable variants accessible to human psychobiology" (Marshall 1985, vii), he has formulated (Marshall 1982, 165) four "constraints to which effective orthography must conform." These are requirements on ease of discrimination, execution, learning, and deciphering the written code. Note that no linguistic terms are introduced. This, it seems, is no accident. The analogy Marshall makes between Universal Grammar and the universal orthographic code is dubious. There are reasons to believe that significant universal generalizations over writing systems are not possible. First, these systems developed subsequent to language. Second, they were consciously designed by humans. Third, they are taught by explicit instruction, and not learned spontaneously. Fourth, there are observable individual differences among poor and good readers. On each of these measures, spoken language gives the opposite result. It is thus not surprising that Marshall's functional characterization consists of psychobiological constraints on design of a very general nature and has little to do with structural (phonological) variables. It is difficult to see how a statement of grapheme-to-phoneme conversion rules can be made, based on the principles Marshall proposes. Thus, even if we accepted the universal principles he offers, we would still be in need of a phonology-based explication of the "grapheme-to-phoneme conversion" process.

3. *The domains of information-processing models are arbitrarily selected.* Many information-processing models are designed to account for linguistic and other *activities,* as opposed to mental structures. And as Fodor and Garrett put it very clearly in the paragraph quoted earlier, what cognitive science should concentrate on is the latter, not the former. It is not clear, for instance, why Patterson and Coltheart (as well as others) choose the five dimensions listed earlier as criteria for reading performance. Although these tests provide a clinical classification of patients, there is no guarantee that it is the relevant classification for understanding the reading process. As another example, consider models proposed for number recognition (Caramazza and McCloskey 1985) and for reading, writing, and repetition (Caramazza, Miceli, and Villa 1986, 82). These aim "to formulate a detailed model of a particular cognitive system which when 'lesioned' appropriately functions in such a way as to generate the patterns of cognitive impairments observed in brain-damaged patients" (Caramazza, Miceli, and Villa 1986, 82). Though in principle this is a reasonable approach, the selection of the domain is totally unmotivated: it seems quite unlikely that there is a special processor in the human head that is designed specifically to read Arabic numbers and convert them into spoken phoneme sequences, or that there is a special repetition device. The standard evolutionary arguments suggest that such an independent "cognitive module" is quite unlikely to exist. Rather, it is much more likely that activities like this are supported by a processor responsible for much more. There are quite convincing arguments for the existence of an independent "language organ" in the human mind (see, for example, Chomsky 1980), as well as for visual and auditory modules (Fodor 1983). But in the present case, unless reasons are given for the existence of a separate subprocessor (or a distinct knowledge system) for numbers, there is no reason to believe that activities like number recognition or repetition are more than epiphenomena; they seem to be derived (or "piggybacked" on some other systems, to use a term suggested by Edgar Zurif). Loss of those abilities is not sufficient evidence for the existence of independent underlying processors.

4. *Information-processing systems are unconstrained.* No constraints are imposed on the internal structure of these models, and processors and subprocessors and subsubprocessors can proliferate endlessly. As a result, this approach is merely ad hoc and does little more than restate the data it wishes to explain. A different methodology is needed (for more on this issue see Zurif, Swinney, and Garrett, in press).[5]

1.3.3 Neurological Constraints on Theories of Language Knowledge and Use

The critique of the connectionist and information-processing approaches, in conjunction with the changes that have taken place in linguistics and psycholinguistics, leads quite naturally to the approach taken here. Given the view of language users as possessing grammars that help them produce, comprehend, read, and write linguistic expressions in their language, I will propose an analysis of language deficits that adheres to models in which attention is paid not just to channels through which language can be practiced but also to its structural properties. I will show that important insights concerning the structure, processing, and acquisition of the linguistic signal can be gained by looking at aphasic syndromes.

To expand on the structure of the argument in this book and how it links neuropsychological data to theoretical questions in linguistics and psycholinguistics: In general, a theory is said to explain a set of facts if they are deducible from it. In the chapters that follow several theoretical frameworks will be put to an empirical test. Linguistic, psycholinguistic, and potentially other theories that are of interest to cognitive scientists will be held accountable not just for normal data but also for impairment patterns in cognitive deficits. On this view, data from grammaticality judgments of normal speakers (the standard object of explanation in linguistics) are no different in status from acquisition data, reaction time data obtained by psycholinguistic experimentation, or data from aphasia, as long as an explicit mapping is given between the observed performance and the theory. Many claims of this type have been made in the past, yet many are faulty precisely in this respect (see chapter 4). The method used here, then, will differ from both connectionism and information processing in that rather than looking at linguistic activities and processes, it will take into account the structural properties of the linguistic signal. It further contrasts with connectionism in that it makes no claims concerning the relation between mental processes and neural tissue.

The procedure used repeatedly throughout the book is this: It begins with an examination of a data set, taken from one theoretically defined cognitive domain. A descriptive framework is chosen to state generalizations over these data. Predictions are derived concerning further patterns of impairment and sparing, forcing reformulation and refinement of the theoretical characterization of the deficit in question, and extending the data base. Finally, the description obtained is used to motivate constraints on a class of theories: they are required to have the property that the descriptive generalization over the pathological data can be stated without adding any ad hoc machinery to them. That is, the patterns of selectivity in the relevant domain observed after brain damage have to form *natural classes* in the theory. The internal structure of the theoretical account of a domain, then, effectively dictates which patterns of impairment are possible, and which are impossible. An examination of deficit descriptions can be used to evaluate the theory. If the predictions it makes are correct, and it is found to be compatible with breakdown patterns, we can conclude that it meets the neuropsychological constraint of *breakdown-compatibility*. This will be added to two other proposed constraints on the theory of grammar: those of *learnability* and *parsability*.

The view of language deficits as disruptions that may be described along grammatical as well as channel lines has some interesting implications. Take the notion "pure case," for instance. This is how traditional neurological studies characterize their ideal finding: a patient suffering impairment to one activity, whereas all the others are intact. (For example, pure alexia is loss of the ability to read, with every other mental capacity unharmed.) Traditional neurological models sought pure losses of a variety of language-related activities to buttress a view of language as an aggregate of dissociable capacities to engage in these activities. For them, a pure case isolated one "atom" in their theory, and since their units of analysis were the various linguistic activities, brain damage could not cut the cognitive pie in a manner finer than these. But in the present context, where the mode through which language is practiced is just a part of the story, the notion "pure case" is interpreted differently. In this context, we can imagine the breakdown of a *part* of each activity, that is, a disruption either to processes underlying activity through a given channel or to knowledge underlying all channels. Hence, accepting the validity of theories of mental representation leads us to neuropsychological accounts that are sensitive to both channel and linguistic elements.

One more comment concerning theoretical accounts of cognitive deficits: If one is interested only in a precise description of observed deficits, one need not be concerned with constructing a unique account. There can be more than one way (and one theory) to accommodate a given pattern. The question of uniqueness arises only if the aim is to constrain normal theories. For this purpose, it must be shown that the properties of a deficit description that are claimed to motivate the constraint are not the result of the arbitrary selection of a theoretical framework. Alternative formulations must be ruled out in this case; otherwise, the constraint does not follow. That is, it must be demonstrated that the result obtained is not an accidental consequence of the particular theory chosen to describe the phenomena but instead that it holds generally.

As an example, consider the pathologies that tend to cluster around agrammatic aphasia. It is generally acknowledged that hemiplegia to the side contralateral to the dominant hemisphere is frequently associated with agrammatic aphasia (Geschwind 1965; Mohr 1976), yet no sensible psychologically oriented description of the syndrome would include hemiplegia as a significant pathognomonic or would claim that the linguistic impairment follows from the same underlying mechanism that derives the hemiplegia. Indeed, most accounts contend that the two pathologies cooccur merely because of the accidental anatomic proximity of the motor strip to the speech area and not because the same neural machinery underlies both motor and linguistic behavior.[6] Similarly, if one's interests are, say, in syntax, and if syntax is assumed to be distinct from phonology in a well-defined way, then the description of syntactic patterns of loss and sparing in a syndrome should be distinct from (yet not incompatible with) the description of the impaired phonology.

Criticisms of such statements as "not capturing all the data at hand" (a common formula) must always be both met with caution and taken with a grain of salt. On the one hand, one would ideally like them to be as general as possible. On the other, it should be acknowledged that a cluster of cognitive aberrations caused by a physical agent (such as a stroke) does not necessarily lend itself to a uniform description, and even if it does, a generalization is always in danger of being spurious. This is true for any scientific domain, and for neuropsychology in particular, even if what is at issue is a set of behaviors caused by a single event. In describing a deficit, I intend no "comprehensive" characterization of the impairment or definition of a syndrome. Like virtually every student of neuropsychological disturbances, I will focus on those aspects of the pathology that will be relevant to the question of interest and ignore all the rest. I will thus abstract away from many observed behavioral aberrations, as is commonly done.

At every point, it is the investigator's task to determine how far descriptive generalizations can be carried—a task that sometimes turns out to be extremely difficult. In the chapters that follow I discuss and criticize several such descriptions, propose and defend a new one, and point out its merits and shortcomings.

The theories to be considered are all connected to language. They concern linguistic knowledge that humans possess (theories of syntax), the way this knowledge is used (psycholinguistic models and theories of language perception), and the manner by which this knowledge develops (models of language acquisition). The concentration on language follows from the focus on aphasic deficits, and the patterns of selective impairment they exhibit, as the main source of data.

Imposing neurologically based constraints on linguistic theories is a central— yet not the only—goal of this book. I will also argue that cognitive deficits offer us a special view of our mental life. The inability to utilize some processes might shed light on others and enable us to discover processes that could not be discovered through observations on neurologically intact individuals. Aphasic syndromes open this type of a special possibility for those interested in the processors underlying our linguistic abilities. If some of a speaker's linguistically relevant resources are blocked, certain other, rarely used processes show up; we can examine their interaction with the remains of the language processor and thereby learn about its internal structure. Specifically, I will argue that the language processor is modular, in that the flow of information between it and other parts of the cognitive system is severely restricted. I will demonstrate this by examining the manner in which nonlinguistic knowledge interacts with linguistic knowledge following brain damage.

Finally, I will examine the relation between two states where humans exhibit partial linguistic ability: language acquisition and language deficit. I will argue that we can motivate analogies between patterns of breakdown and patterns of acquisition, albeit in a rather limited way.

In sum, the relation between neuropsychological disorders and cognitive theories is bidirectional. On the one hand, theories are used as *discovery procedures* for the deficits. On the other, impairment patterns are used to motivate *constraints* on the internal structure of the theories and to obtain unique clues about the internal structure of the mechanisms underlying normal cognitive capacities.

1.4   On Studying Behavioral Aberrations Whose Cause Is Physical

1.4.1   On Error Analysis

I have been talking about behavioral aberrations all along. It is time now to discuss their nature and the logic of investigations into such phenomena. In the domains we are concerned with, *errors* form the main type of aberration.[7] The cognitively relevant disturbances are errors of identification and recognition (Warrington and Taylor 1973; Etcoff 1984; Yin 1970), errors of movement (Heilman 1979), production of ungrammatical strings, miscomprehension, and abnormal judgment of grammaticality. Such phenomena are interesting because patterns that can be observed in erroneous performances might give clues about the normal system. A first step in this direction is to state a descriptive generalization over these patterns, by a modified normal model. The crucial question is, What is the nature of such modifications?

A first piece of an answer comes from J. A. Fodor (1985), whose observation concerning a peculiar dilemma actually helps in clarifying things for us. In his discussion of the nature of causal explanation in representational theories of mind, he considers how one can build up a theory that will also allow for occasional erroneous performance. After all, people make errors from time to time, and a good theory must allow this to happen. He presents the following dilemma (which he calls "the disjunction problem"). Suppose, he says, that in our causal explanation the represented symbol 'A' is such that its tokens are caused by things A (or things having the property A, and so on). Then 'A' tokens are *always* caused by A's. But to allow for error, there must be some B that is causally related to 'A' tokening. In this case 'A' would be a misrepresentation of B, and error would be possible.

The problem is that if 'A' tokens are caused by A's and B's (and this is the situation now, since misrepresentation is permitted), then 'A' tokens are not caused reliably by A's but instead are caused disjunctively by ($B \vee A$). But in this case 'A' tokens caused by B are no longer misrepresentations. Rather, they are part and parcel of the explanation. The theory no longer admits error.

Here is another way of putting it. According to Fodor, a representational theory of mind should account for those occasional instances where upon being confronted with a horse, we mistakenly construct a representation of a motorcycle. But if we assume that a representation of 'MOTORCYCLE' is invoked by both motorcycles and horses, then these occasional instances are no longer errors ("wild" tokenings, in Fodor's terms) but instead are causally explained. Tokens of 'MOTORCYCLE' are now caused by exposure to either horses or motorcycles.

Fodor then considers possible solutions. For us, however, the very presentation of the dilemma would suffice, for it sheds light on the nature of our explanation of behavioral aberrations of the type we are interested in. In particular, although our focus is on misrepresentation, it is not on misrepresentation of the usual kind. We are not talking about occasional errors. Rather, we are talking about systematic error patterns that, for all practical purposes, are due to an identifiable physical cause and that reoccur reliably over time. We are thus concerned with the proper representation of reliable misrepresentation, so to speak. It is this goal that distinguishes our enterprise from the one that emerges from Fodor's dilemma. For us, yesterday's abnormality (the error by our standards) is today's norm (the patient's stable performance).

What does our modified normal theory do for us? We want to know what went wrong with our brain-damaged subject. We are looking for a causal explanation that is based on a normal model. We have two options. We can assume that some knowledge, processes, or mechanisms were lost and show how the remaining mental faculty behaves the way it does—how the spared components interact and underlie the aberrant behavior. Alternatively, we can assume that a faculty was completely destroyed and that its function was taken over by some other functional system. Various considerations such as parsimony and descriptive adequacy point to the former possibility in the context of the cognitive deficit to be analyzed. Importantly, we are committed to a causal explanation of what went wrong, and exactly how someone could be normal on Sunday, and from Monday on produce errors like those we observe for the patients. And for an explanation like this we must assume that normal individuals *never* make mistakes in the domains in question—that their faculty is impeccable—and that the mistakes we see in them are caused by some agent, which must be a part of our explanation.

This type of account has two advantages. First, since we are to modify a normal model, and since the choice of model determines the range of possible modifications, we can evaluate normal theories by their modifiability. Second, since we will have to introduce new, normally unobserved factors into the explanation, we will have a rare chance to take a look at the back side of our mind.

1.4.2   On Relating Brain Damage and Behavioral Aberration
The next questions we should consider are these: What are the primitives of our account, and what kinds of statements should count as explanatory in our context?

One way of thinking about cognitively impaired humans is as participants in a controlled psychological experiment: they are under some conditions in which some of their capacities cannot be expressed. There is one difference, however: most experimentally induced conditions are created by manipulating the environment or the stimulus, whereas in the case of cognitive impairment it is the tissue subserving the mental faculty in question that is damaged.[8] This immediately begs a question concerning the nature of the best account of the behavioral patterns observed in the deficit. Unlike standard experimental manipulations, this one is caused internally, by identifiable physical agents. Should we, then, explain the behavioral aberration by referring to neuroanatomical terms?

In my opinion, the answer is no. If one accepts some version of the representational theory of mind, then mental events are not reducible to physical events (for convincing arguments, see Fodor 1975, 1981). A fortiori, mental aberrations are not reducible to physical aberrations; that is, an assertion such as "Jones is aphasic because the left half of his brain is missing" does not count as a psychological explanation, even though it might be observationally true. (In fact, even for an identity theorist, who would equate brain states with mental states, this kind of statement is far from constituting a sufficient explanation.) More intuitively, think about, say, the language faculty, the neural tissue supporting it, and the vessels supplying it with blood. Acquired language disorders are most commonly observed after damage to one of the blood vessels. Does that mean that the cerebral arrangement of these vessels is a determinant of our linguistic abilities? The answer here is categorically no.

There are different levels of understanding for the description of the activities subserved by neural tissue, and mental operations underlying linguistic behavior are certainly many levels apart from physical entities like blood vessels. (See Marr and Poggio 1977 for a well-articulated argument to that effect, with an example from the visual system.) The building blocks for cognitive deficit descriptions therefore come from cognitive theories, and it is just these theories to which neuropsychological phenomena—at the psychological level of description—are relevant. This obvious point is not accepted by many—specifically, those belonging to the "localizationist" school. (See Ojemann 1983 for an extreme position, and Grodzinsky 1985 for a critique of this approach.) These investigators identify mental faculties (which are usually defined quite arbitrarily) with specific cerebral loci. Yet these two entities are many levels apart, and to associate them directly amounts to a category mistake.

1.5   Toward an Application of the Argument: Forecast

So far I have presented my approach to cognitive deficits in a general fashion. I have argued for it without really giving an illustration, and I have given reasons to believe that other approaches are faulty. In the remainder of this book I provide empirical support for my arguments.

I begin with descriptive issues. In chapter 2 I sketch the theoretical framework that I will use throughout the book. I review the main themes and principles of current syntactic theory, as presented in Chomsky 1981 and various later works. In this review I emphasize those aspects of the theory that are directly relevant for the discussions to follow, at times sacrificing precision for clarity. In chapter 3 I consider agrammatism. I take the reader on a tour through clinical features, experimental findings, and past approaches and then make several proposals of my own, examining agrammatism from a formal linguistic perspective. I show that it is a deficit that is closely tied to grammar in both production and comprehension and that it is therefore very relevant to language-related cognitive theories. Once I have precisely characterized this syndrome, I use the characterization to inform cognitive theories in the manner described earlier. In chapter 4 I look at linguistic theories and formulate neurologically based constraints for them. In chapter 5 I use brain damage to get a unique look at the language processor and to obtain clues concerning its modular structure. Finally, in chapter 6 I discuss questions that arise when neuropsychological issues are confronted with theories of language acquisition.

Chapter 2
The Linguistic Framework

2.1 Introduction

Since the subject matter of this book is aberrant language and its relevance to theories of normal linguistic behavior, it will be helpful at the outset to look at some concepts of current linguistic theory. This chapter is intended to be a convenient reference for the reader not fully familiar with current syntactic concepts. It is not a survey of linguistics, nor is it a thorough review of one theoretical framework. Rather, it presents the aspects of syntax that are used later in the book and provides a general description of the framework in which they are couched: Government-Binding Theory (Chomsky 1981, 1986a, b, and much related literature). [1]

A grammar is a formal definition of a language. It seeks to explain why certain sequences of words constitute well-formed sentences in a language, whereas others do not. Grammatical theory views language as a set, and serves as a membership criterion, where the elements of the set are usually sentences. A grammar is a collection of rules for the formation of well-formed strings. Universal Grammar (UG) is that set of statements that characterizes the universal properties of *grammar*—those properties that, at the right level of abstraction, are found in every grammar of the world's languages and, moreover, in any grammar that humans can conceivably possess. UG, then, is a characterization of the notion "a possible human language."

Several constructs have played a central role in generative grammar since its conception in the 1950s. These are the notions "level of representation," "lexicon," "phrase structure rule," and "transformation." A transformational generative grammar of the 1950s and 1960s typically consisted of two levels of representation (Surface structure and Deep structure), a lexicon that served as a source for elements (words and their properties), recursive phrase structure rules that generated structural descriptions (tree structures) for strings, and transformations that mapped one level onto the other. Deep structure was the syntax-semantics interface, and Surface structure connected with phonology. The similarity in meaning between, say, active and passive sentences was explained by assuming that the phrase structure rules generated the same Deep structure representation for both, which was in fact the tree structure for the active. This representation was altered by a transformation that changed the order of constituents and added passive morphology and *by* to derive the passive. A question was derived transformationally from the corresponding declarative by replacing the element to be questioned with a *wh*-word and moving the wh-word to the front of the sentence. The grammar consisted of a list of phrase structure rules, responsible for the basic syntactic structures of a language (all the Deep structure configurations) and several transformations—rules for changing the order of constituents, each stated with a specification of its domain of application (its structural description). Only sentences that could be derived by this rule system counted as grammatical. Presentations of such theories can be found in Chomsky 1957, 1965.

Yet linguists soon realized that such rule systems would not suffice. If the theory says that the passive transformation can be applied in an unrestricted fashion, then why can't it apply twice?

(1) a. John hit Bill.
     b. Bill was hit (by John).
     c. Mary said that John hit Bill.
     d. Mary said that Bill was hit (by John).
     e. *Bill was said that was hit (by John) (by Mary).

Alternatively, why is it impossible to form questions in some contexts?

(2) a. Mary said that John hit Bill.
     b. Who did Mary say John hit?
     c. Mary told the story that John hit Bill.
     d. *Who did Mary tell the story that John hit?

These issues, as well as others, led to a change in approach. It turned out that rule systems that characterize grammars are highly constrained—that in order to achieve descriptive adequacy, the manner in which transformations and other rules apply must be limited. Theoreticians shifted their focus to the study of these constraints, believing them to be the locus of the real universal principles underlying natural language. Moreover, since languages vary, it was proposed that constraints should be stated parametrically. The Italian equivalent of sentence (2d), for example, is grammatical. This cross-linguistic difference can be captured if we assume a constraint that prohibits questioning in certain contexts in English but in others in Italian (see Rizzi 1982). Thus, linguistic theory is currently concerned with parametrically formulated principles that constrain rule systems and guarantee the well-formedness of representations. The principles are organized in modules, each consisting of one or more statements. The interaction of the different modules tightly constrains possible representations. What follows is a brief presentation of this theory, with emphasis on the parts that are relevant to this work.

2.2   The T-Model and Its Modular Organization

Generative theories of grammar have posited several representations associated with each sentence in a given language. In its current incarnation, Government-Binding (GB) Theory posits four: D-structure (corresponding roughly to Deep structure of earlier models), S-structure (somewhat similar to Surface structure), Phonetic Form (PF) (representing phenomena associated with the phonology-syntax interface), and Logical Form (LF) (where issues of scope, quantification, and the like are handled). The organization of the grammar is given in figure 2.1.

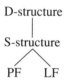

Figure 2.1

The modularly organized principles apply to representations at the various levels. Each module has its designated domain. That is, the principles of grammar do not necessarily all apply at all levels. Some (such as X' theory—read "X-bar theory"—which constrains phrase structure) apply at D-structure; some (such as Case theory) apply at S-structure; some apply at other levels; and one principle—the Projection Principle—applies at all levels of representation. The modules (in boxes) and their domains (indicated by arrows) are illustrated in figure 2.2.

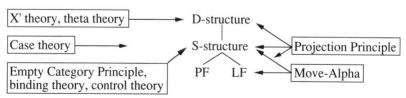

Figure 2.2

A sentence is well formed just in case its representations at all levels are well formed, that is, if it satisfies all the constraints everywhere. When well-formedness is defined this way, the need for rules is reduced. If previous types of generative grammars had to generate all the grammatical strings of a language, and only those, the phrase structure and transformational rules of this type of grammar can generate freely (and optimally permit the generation of any sequence of elements), producing both grammatical and ungrammatical sequences. The constraints stated in the theory rule out ungrammatical monsters and thus ensure that only the grammatical sentences end up in the language. So, for example, rather than formulating many transformational rules—one for passive sentences, one for questions, and so on—we may now state a very general rule—Move-Alpha, a transformation that can basically move anything anywhere—and rely on the constraints to rule out bad derivations. The sections that follow describe the modules in more detail.

2.3   X' Theory and the Lexicon

A grammar of a given language contains phrase structure rules that characterize the range of possible structures in the language. But what kinds of rules are possible? Could we imagine a language, for instance, that has rules like those in (3)?

(3)   a.   NP → P VP
      b.   VP → NP S
      c.   N → VP

Such rules do not exist in the grammars of natural languages. Yet in the first formulations of the theory there was nothing to exclude them. So, just like the need for constraints on movement rules, there arose a need for a general characterization of possible phrase structure rules, a characterization that would restrict in advance the range of possibilities. This led various investigators to propose X' theory (Chomsky 1970; Jackendoff 1977; Stowell 1981), which provides general schemas for possible phrase structure rule types and which later turned out to have other advantages.

Central to the schema are the traditional notions "head," "complement," and "projection." A head is a linguistic unit or element that gives a larger unit its character. Heads are found in more than one category. Thus, a noun is the head of a noun phrase, and a verb is the head of a verb phrase. In general, every major lexical category (N, V, A, P) heads a phrase, and this phrase is a projection of that category. In addition to a head, a phrase may contain a complement—element(s) that the head subcategorizes for. For example, a noun may subcategorize for a sentence (4a); a verb may subcategorize for a noun phrase (4b); and so on.

(4) a. the claim [that John is stupid]
     b. hit [Bill]

A phrase may also contain modifiers and specifiers. The hierarchical ordering among these elements motivates the assumption that a phrase has several levels. It follows that a phrase contains more than one projection: a zero projection X (lexical categories N, V, A, P), intermediate projections, and a maximal projection X^{max} (in our case, NP, VP, and so on). It is commonly assumed that the maximal number is two. The generalized schema is illustrated in (5).

(5)   X'' (maximal projection)

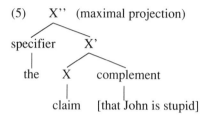

This schema is a cross-categorial constraint, so every phrase structure rule must abide by it. Rules such as those in (3) cannot be stated in such a framework. The schema, then, constrains the grammar, for it limits the range of possible rules and excludes those that are not encountered anywhere. In fact, some current versions of GB Theory do not even state phrase structure rules. They permit the generation of any tree, and let X' theory and other principles in the various modules rule out whatever does not satisfy them. The claim (or rather, the desideratum) is that the principles are stated so precisely that they suffice to distinguish good from bad strings and structural descriptions.

Having discussed the rules for the construction of phrase structure, we should now look at the building blocks of strings in the language—the words—and the way they are represented in the grammar. Words are contained in the lexicon—an indispensable source of information for a grammar. As models of generative grammar have grown more sophisticated, the role of the lexicon has increased. If in the beginning words were derived by simple phrase structure rules that expanded lexical categories into words, just like an expansion of an S into an NP VP sequence, then today there is much more information and structure in the lexicon. It stores idiosyncratic facts about individual words, yet there are certain important generalizations regarding its internal structure. Central to it are the concepts of argument structure and subcategorization, which are types of information it encodes.

Words of the same category differ with respect to the syntactic and semantic properties of their complements. For example, a verb may take from zero to two nominal complements (6a–c) and may also have a sentential (6d) or prepositional (6e) complement.

(6) a. John slept.
   b. John saw Bill.
   c. John gave Bill a picture.
   d. John said that Bill left.
   e. John believed in God.

These facts must be encoded somehow, to avoid deriving strings that would fit verbs with inappropriate structures.

(7) a. *John slept Bill.
   b. *John saw Bill a picture.
   c. *John gave that Bill left.
   d. *John said Bill.
   e. *John believed.

Different words also take arguments that play different semantic roles. For example, the subject of *give*, functioning as a source of action, plays a semantic role different from that of the subject of *adore*, functioning as an experiencer of an event. The lexicon, then, encodes the number of arguments a lexical item is associated with, their syntactic categories, and the roles they play (their thematic labels). A word in the lexicon is thus associated with a subcategorization frame and with the labels of the thematic (roughly semantic) roles played by the arguments it selects, written in its thematic grid.[2] Rules that apply to an item in the lexicon must take all these facts into account. So although there may be a rule of the form in (8a), it cannot be applied to the element in (8b), because of the mismatch in the number of arguments.

(8) a. VP→V NP NP
   b. hit: [__ NP]
   c. *John hit Bill Mary.

With all the information built into the system so far, we do not yet have a device that blocks derivations such as (8c). We need an explicit requirement that will ensure the match in properties between the lexical entry and the rule. To this end, the *Projection Principle* has been devised. This principle, of which Chomsky's (1981, 29) formulation is given in (9), guarantees that idiosyncrasies of lexical entries are honored throughout the grammar.

(9) *Projection Principle*
   Representations at each syntactic level are projected from the lexicon, in that they observe the subcategorization properties of lexical items.

The Projection Principle is a very important element of GB Theory. It not only ensures that lexical categories are not concatenated with elements for which they are not subcategorized but also constrains the mapping from D-structure to S-structure. If the D-structure representation of a sentence contains an NP position, then that position must be represented at the level of S-structure, too, even if a transformational rule that applied to move constituents around has vacated a position. As we will see, this forces the assumption that there are syntactically represented positions that are actually devoid of phonetic content (empty categories).

2.4   Move-Alpha, Traces, and Subjacency

The notion of a transformation has always been central to generative grammar. It was recognized that regularities of certain types must be expressed by rules that not only establish hierarchy among sentential constituents but also represent other kinds of dependencies that hold among syntactic positions. To this end, a particular type of mapping from Deep to Surface structure was assumed, one that takes strings, substitutes elements in them, and adjoins or deletes others. Initially a large number of transformations were assumed, some obligatory and some optional. Yet since this arrangement presents an enormous task to language learners, who are forced not only to learn many rules but also to know which are obligatory and which are optional, efforts have been made to reduce the number of transformational rules. As noted earlier, this can be done by stating just one rule, very generally, and positing constraints on its application (or, alternatively, on the well-formedness of the representations it can output). Therefore, rather than assuming one transformation to derive passive sentences, one to derive questions, and so on, GB theorists now assume one rule—Move-Alpha—which may move anything anywhere. This rule, importantly, is optional. Other principles are expected to sift away undesirable results.

Let us now examine how Move-Alpha interacts with other subcomponents of the grammar. Move-Alpha is a mapping operation that can delete or substitute categories. It follows that passivization, for example, consists of deleting an NP that is in object position in D-structure and substituting that NP for the subject. But the Projection Principle is stated to guarantee that lexical requirements are met at every level. Therefore, if a verb selects an NP as its object, deleting that NP would violate the Projection Principle. To avoid that, GB theorists assume that movement may result in a phonologically empty yet structurally represented position, filled with a construct called a *trace*. The trace is further linked to the moved NP (its antecedent) by a common index. (We will see that this coindexing has important uses.) The operation of Move-Alpha is exemplified in (10).

(10) a.   [e] was hit [John]   (D-structure)
     b.   [John]$_i$ was hit t$_i$ (S-structure)

The distribution of traces has been studied extensively over the past few years. What used to be different movement rules (most notably, Move-*Wh* and Move-*NP*) are now collapsed into Move-Alpha, yet the properties of the traces of the different movement types are distinct. Given the modular organization of the grammar, it is easy to see how different well-formedness conditions may apply to the different types of traces. A *wh*-trace, for instance, behaves like a logical variable (the question *Who did John meet?* may be interpreted as 'for which person x, John met x'), whereas an NP-trace (in passive and Raising) does not. Also, a *wh*-trace has Case (see section 2.6), whereas an NP-trace does not. Thus, the fact that the grammar has several subcomponents allows the rules to be stated very generally and still leaves room for descriptively necessary distinctions, which are now made through the interplay of the modules.

A trace and its antecedent are linked, and this connection is captured by the concept *syntactic chain*. A chain is a representation of all the elements that share a mutual index, which they acquired through movement. As we will see, this is a useful construct: certain syntactic processes (mainly thematic marking) are best defined over chains. The relationship between the trace and its antecedent is governed by *Subjacency*, a constraint whose task is to rule out ungrammatical strings like (2d), which resulted from a transformational operation that moved a constituent "too far." The permissible distance is defined over tree structures— a moved constituent cannot cross more than one node with a particular label— and the category types that block movement vary from language to language. This is a clear case of parametric variation: the same general principle is stated universally, but the details vary cross-linguistically.

In sum, then, Move-Alpha is a general movement rule that leaves a trace behind, and Subjacency is a condition on movement.

2.5   The Theta Criterion, Theta Theory, and Government

We have seen that the lexicon contains varied information. Among other things, a word's lexical entry encodes the number and content of the arguments that are associated with that word. This is the word's *thematic grid* (Stowell 1981), where each position of an argument is labeled with a *thematic (theta) role* (although we will see that some linguists have questioned this assumption). Also needed, for interpretation, are (1) a process by which theta-roles are assigned and (2) general conditions that guarantee proper assignment. For that the *Theta* Criterion has been devised, a condition that is closely related to the Projection Principle. Before discussing it, however, we should look at the motivation for thematic relations (and the whole thematic module).

The notion of thematic relations was first introduced in generative grammar by Gruber (1965). These relations, which are presumably drawn from a small universal inventory, identify roles that arguments play with respect to a predicate. Each predicate has a set of such roles associated with it, and their assignment to arguments is guided and constrained by a set of universal principles. Central to Gruber's system (which was further developed in Jackendoff's (1972) seminal monograph) is the notion of *theme*, which, by hypothesis, is present in every predicate-argument structure. The sentences in (11) illustrate the notion, covering the roles that are considered central.

(11) a. John hit Bill.
       agent   theme

   b. Fred slept.
     theme

   c. Mary received a present from Mark.
     goal   theme   source

   d. Sue put the book on the desk.
     agent   theme   location

   e. John admired Mary.
     experiencer theme

Since these roles have a semantic flavor (having labels that correspond to semantic functions), the question immediately arises whether there is a need for such constructs in a theory of syntax that distinguishes itself from semantic theory. Jackendoff (1987) presents the argument that convinced him of this need, since it shows that some syntactic problems cannot be solved without making reference to thematic relations.

(12) a. John$_i$ gave Sue$_j$ orders PRO$_j$ to leave.
   b. John$_i$ got from Sue$_j$ orders PRO$_i$ to leave.
   c. John$_i$ gave Sue$_j$ a promise PRO$_i$ to leave.
   d. John$_i$ got from Sue$_j$ a promise PRO$_j$ to leave.

The problem, Jackendoff points out, "is that these are all structurally identical in the relevant respects [they have the same phrase marker], so there is no apparent syntactic condition that determines the antecedent of PRO [an abstract representation of the "logical" subject of the infinitive]" (p. 369).

Yet if one attaches theta-role labels to the arguments according to what each deverbal noun dictates, the story changes, since it is always the goal of order (Sue in (12a), John in (12b)), and the source of the promise (John in (12c), Sue in

(12d))who would have to leave a fact which makes it the antecedent of PRO. A syntactic fact that cannot be explained otherwise is thus accounted for, and the need for thematic relations as syntactic constructs is justified.

Since the appearance of Gruber's and Jackendoff's original work, much research has been done on thematic relations. In fact, they have come to play a central role in linguistic theory in recent years. Since the introduction of the Theta Criterion (Chomsky 1981), the notion of theta-grid (Stowell 1981), and the attempt to eliminate phrase structure rules from the theory, much effort has been put into specifying the inventory of thematic relations, their exact role, the manner by which they are represented for each predicate, the rules that link them to arguments, and the general principles that constrain these rules. For instance, a famous principle that encoded theta-roles to account for syntactic facts is the Thematic Hierarchy Condition (Jackendoff 1972). This principle was formulated to explain why some verbs passivize, whereas others do not.

(13) a. John paid two dollars (for the potatoes).
        | |
      agent   theme

    b. The potatoes cost two dollars.
          | |
       theme   location

    c. Two dollars were paid by John (for the potatoes).

    d. *Two dollars were cost by the potatoes.

Jackendoff proposed that a universal hierarchy holds among theta-roles and that the order of theta-roles in sentences is constrained by this hierarchy.

(14) *Thematic Hierarchy*
    1. Agent
    2. Location, source, goal
    3. Theme

Thematic Hierarchy Condition (THC)
    The passive *by*-phrase must be higher on the Thematic Hierarchy than the derived subject.

The asymmetries in (13) are thus explained. Passivization of (13a) results in a well-formed structure, where the by-phrase contains agent and theme is the derived subject; yet passivization of (13b) would violate the THC because location (which is used rather abstractly in this context) is higher on the Thematic Hierarchy than theme, which will be in the by-phrase.

The THC is one example of how thematic relations can do important syntactic work. Jackendoff and others have proposed extensions to it, and in the past few years thematic relations have been harnessed to the effort to reduce the number of rules and rule types that constitute the theory of syntax. Lexical entries of nouns and verbs thus consist of lists of such roles, known as theta-grids, illustrated in (15); and a general principle ensures a one-to-one relation between arguments that appear in the syntactic representation and those that are listed in the grid (16).

(15) put: <agent, theme, location>

(16) *Theta Criterion* (Chomsky 1981)
    Each argument in a sentence is associated with one (and only one) theta-role; each theta-role is associated with one (and only one) argument.

The Theta Criterion thus ensures congruence between theta-roles and positions in the sentence. The assignment of theta-roles (theta-marking) is subject to *government* (a structural relation that must hold between assigner and assignee), whose definition (or, rather, one version of it) is given in (17).

(17) *Government*
    α governs γ in the structure [$_\beta$...γ...α...γ...] where,
    a. $\alpha = X^0$
    b.   where ϕ is a maximal projection, ϕ dominates γ if and only if ϕ dominates α.

A question immediately arises: If theta-marking takes place under government, and if predicates assign theta-roles to their arguments in a fixed manner, then what happens to moved constituents? Where does the subject of the passive, for instance, get its theta-role from? Two types of theta-marking are thus distinguished: direct and indirect. A verb always assigns a theta-role to the same position, regardless of its phonetic content. If that position is filled with a "real" NP, then theta-marking is direct. If it is occupied by a trace, then theta-marking is indirect: the theta-role is assigned to the trace, which then transmits that role to its antecedent. Given that these two constitute a chain, it follows that a chain is assigned one theta-role only. Like other modules of the grammar, Theta theory involves parametric variation, since the direction of theta-role assignment may vary: in some languages theta-roles are assigned from right to left, and in others they are assigned from left to right. This may be (and in fact has been) used to account for cross-linguistic differences in word order (see, for example, Travis 1984).

Two major debates currently dominate the literature on thematic relations. First, do syntactic rules refer to thematic *labels,* or is it enough to refer merely to the *number* of such roles? Second, do arguments contained in thematic representations participate in any ordering relationships (hierarchical or not), or do they constitute simply an unordered list?

Concerning the first issue, one view is that certain syntactic generalizations cannot be expressed without referring directly to thematic labels (see, for example, Jackendoff 1987). The opposing view denies this need (see, for example, Grimshaw, forthcoming; Levin and Rappaport 1986). In chapter 3 I will show that certain patterns of performance observed in aphasia can be explained only if we refer to thematic labels explicitly (that is, by their content—agent, patient, theme, and so on). Concerning the issue of hierarchy among arguments, again, some authors claim that such a relation exists (Grimshaw, forthcoming), whereas others deny it (Levin and Rappaport 1986).

2.6 Case Theory

Case theory specifies the structural positions in which lexical NPs may appear. The core assumption is that abstract Case (which may or may not have phonetically overt realization) must be assigned to every lexical NP. Certain elements are designated assigners, most notably the inflection on tensed verbs, verbs, and prepositions. It follows that an NP position without Case can contain only an NP-trace. Case theory thus inheres in the *Case Filter*.

(18) *Case Filter*
$$*NP_{[+lexical, -Case]}$$
All lexical NPs must have Case.

To illustrate with an example from the passive construction: Recall that it was assumed that in the formation of a passive sentence Move-Alpha takes the object from D-structure and moves it to the empty subject position. But since Move-Alpha is an optional rule, it does not have to apply, and we could therefore end up with a representation such as (19) at S-structure.

(19) [e] was hit John

This, of course, must be excluded. Therefore, passivization (the conversion of a verb into its passive form) is assumed to consist, among other things, of "Case absorption." A passivized verb no longer assigns Case to its object. Now, given the Case Filter, the object is "forced" to move; otherwise, the result would be an ungrammatical string. (If *John* remained in object position, it would be a lexical NP without Case.) Thus, although Move-Alpha is an optional rule, it is forced to apply because of the existence of the Case Filter.

This subcomponent of the grammar has other desirable consequences. For example, it accounts for the ungrammaticality of the strings in (20a,c), as compared to (20b,d).

(20) a. *John to be there would be great.
    b. For John to be there would be great.
    c. *the destruction the city
    d. the destruction of the city

In (20a) the verb cannot assign Case to *John*, because it is not tensed, hence the ungrammaticality. The appearance of the preposition *for* rescues (20b). Similarly, no Case is assigned to *the city* in (20c), and the insertion of *of* changes the grammatical status of the phrase.

The Case Filter, then, has several applications, and its interaction with other modules results in an explanation of a variety of syntactic facts. Since the direction of Case assignment may vary cross-linguistically, Case theory, like Theta theory, is parametric.

2.7   Binding

Case theory regulates the distribution of lexical NPs. But what is responsible for nonlexical ones? The Binding Conditions determine not only the possible relationships between traces and their antecedents but also the distribution of pronouns and anaphors. In this respect, the binding theory states generalizations that distinguish, not between lexical and nonlexical NPs, but among anaphoric, pronominal, and referring expressions. It turns out that the relationship that holds between empty categories and their antecedents is subject to generalizations similar to those that govern anaphora. Binding theory is thus a tripartite typology of categories, with conditions governing their distribution. Anaphors are reflexive and reciprocal pronouns (like *himself* and *each other*) and the empty categories NP-trace and PRO; pronouns are lexical (nonanaphoric) pronouns (like *he* and *him*) and PRO; and referring (R-)expressions are names and definite descriptions (like *John* and *the man*). The Binding Conditions are given in (21), followed by several definitions of relevant structural relations.

(21) *The Binding Conditions*
    A. An anaphor must be bound in its governing category.
    B. A pronoun must be free in its governing category.
    C. An R-expression must be free.

    Bound: α is bound by β if and only if α and β are coindexed, β c-commands α, and β is in an argument position.
C-command: α c-commands β if the first maximal projection dominating α also dominates β, and α does not contain β.

Governing category: The NP or S in which an element is governed is its governing category.

Argument position: A position where an argument may appear in D-structure (namely, subject or object position) is an argument position.

In short, the Binding Conditions guarantee that anaphors have local antecedents and that pronouns and R-expressions do not. The notion of locality is defined by the governing category. There is plenty of room here for parametric variation. We will return to this issue in chapter 6, where we will consider a parametric definition of governing category in relation to language acquisition and dissolution.

The following cases illustrate the operation of the various Binding Conditions. Consider the contrast in (22).

(22) a. *John wanted [$_S$ Mary to wash himself].
     b. John wanted [$_S$ PRO to wash himself].

The anaphor *himself* in (22a) has a local antecedent: the NP *Mary* is within the embedded S. Since it must be locally bound (by Binding Condition A), then *Mary* must be its binder, and ungrammaticality results from the lack of agreement. The situation in (22b) is different, however, because PRO is coindexed with *John*— its controller (by control theory, which will not be discussed). Thus, it agrees with the anaphor, and the sentence is grammatical.

The next example illustrates Binding Condition B.

(23) a. John wanted [$_S$ Mary to wash him].
     b. *John wanted [$_S$ *Mary* to wash *her*].

The italics in (23b) denote a reading in which the pronoun is coreferential with *Mary*. Such a reading is not possible, because the governing category S containing the pronoun also contains a local antecedent (*Mary*); hence, the pronoun is not free. This is a violation of Binding Condition B, and ungrammaticality follows. In (23a), however, the pronoun is free in its local domain (not bound to *Mary*). Thus, the sentence is grammatical—it comports with the binding theory.

These are just a few illustrations of how grammatical principles operate. More details will be given as we go along. Concerning other important parts of GB Theory (notably the Empty Category Principle and control theory, shown in figure 2.2), see the works cited in note 1.

With this presentation of grammatical priciples—which, though brief, should suffice as a general introduction—we are ready to move on to the formal description of agrammatism and its theoretical consequences.

Chapter 3

The Formal Description of Agrammatism

3.1 Preliminaries

Agrammatic aphasia is a set of pathological phenomena that tend to cluster in individuals who have suffered physical damage in Broca's area and its surroundings.[1] The area implicated is shown in figure 3.1.

The etiologies of this syndrome are varied. It may be caused by stroke (affecting the superior division of the middle cerebral artery), intracranial hemorrhage, protrusion wound, tumor, and other physical agents. From a functional point of view, it appears to consist, minimally, in perceptual and productive problems in the language domain, as well as general cognitive problems of varying severity and kinds; there is often an associated hemiplegia to the side contralateral to the damaged hemisphere. As is true of many related deficits, only a description that consists of terms borrowed from more than one theoretical framework can capture all the observed pathological phenomena of agrammatism. This is because agrammatism is a multifaceted syndrome, which

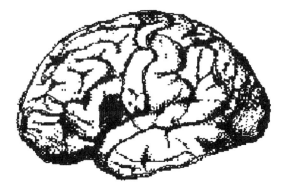

Figure 3.1

seems to impair functioning in more than one cognitive domain—an observation that is not surprising, given that the anatomical organization of cerebral blood vessels is not likely to be sensitive to the functional arrangement of mental faculties. A precise definition of the syndrome (to the extent that it exists) must therefore be based on a cluster of terms. Consequently, when one attempts to account for observed performances from the point of view of some theoretical framework, one must abstract away from many aspects of the data, focusing only on what pertains to the theory in question. Indeed, virtually every descriptive statement found in the literature (and there are many) focuses on *some* aspects of the pathology, namely, those that are believed to have direct relevance to other matters, whether clinical or theoretical.

In the following sections I discuss the proper description of the syntactic deficit in agrammatism. After briefly presenting the "clinical" phenomena, I review previous accounts critically and then propose a new formal characterization of agrammatism, using current theory of grammatical representation as a descriptive procedure. I show that the theory in question is structured in such a way that it conveniently accommodates the agrammatic patterns of selective impairment. In the course of this discussion I abstract away from many aspects of the syndrome (for example, nonfluency in speech and hemiplegia). From the point of view of the descriptive generalization I offer, the cooccurrence of these pathological signs and the rest of the agrammatic phenomena is purely accidental, or at least irrelevant to the theoretical questions I wish to address in later chapters. Their appearance together is related to accidental anatomical proximity to the same blood vessels. Additionally, I consider the description of production and comprehension separately, for reasons that will become apparent later.

3.1.1   Clinical Features
Deleuze reported in 1819 on an aphasic patient who "used exclusively the infinitive of verbs and never used any pronoun. Thus she could say perfectly well, 'Souhaiter bonjour, rester, mari venir'" ('[to] wish good morning, [to] stay, husband [to] come'; see Goodglass and Menn 1985). Later Kussmaul (1876) (cited in Peuser 1978 and Tsvetkova and Glozman 1978) observed brain-damaged patients who showed an "inability to form words grammatically and to arrange phrases syntactically." He called the phenomenon *Akataphasia*. Similarly, Pick (1913) noticed that the production patterns of some Broca's aphasics were aberrant from a grammatical point of view. He did not formulate a precise statement of these speech patterns but simply noted their general abnormality and the fact that word order was largely preserved. He thus argued that such

patients could not construct sentences, even though they seemed to know the "intended preverbal meaning," and termed the phenomenon *agrammatism*.

Currently recognized clinical features of agrammatism are usually found as a part of the description of Broca's aphasia. These consist of nonfluent, effortful speech at a low rate, and poor repetition. The agrammatic manifestation is that "free standing function words and bound morphemes (both inflectional and derivational) often fail to be produced in obligatory contexts" (Marshall 1986, 8). In comprehension, though seemingly normal in a conversational setting, "special testing will usually reveal deficits that seem to parallel the disorder of production" (Marshall 1986, 8).

Over the years there has been some variation among the clinical "definitions" of agrammatism. Goodglass (1968) maintained that "agrammatic patients have a non-fluent speech output consisting of single substantive words or short phrases in which articles, prepositions, personal pronouns, and verb inflections are omitted." Tissot, Mounin, and Lhermitte (1973) listed six defining properties of agrammatism that are accepted as such by most authors. These include a lack of function words, preferred use of substantives, systematic use of infinitives, lack of grammatical agreement, telegraphic style, and the use of stereotypes. Note that these statements refer to speech production patterns only. Now, however, it is acknowledged that the deficits observed in the clinic are actually wider in scope. For instance, Miceli et al. (1983, 66) claim that it is "a general deficit in the patient's ability to utilize grammatical knowledge in both production and comprehension of language. This deficiency is also manifested in both spoken and written modalities." The review and the account below will show that these descriptions are inaccurate.

3.1.2 A Variety of Descriptions

Ever since its discovery, agrammatic aphasia has been the subject of heated debate and the elusive object of descriptive attempts by psychologists, neurologists, and linguists.

Past statements regarding agrammatic phenomena are based on two types of evidence: observations in the clinical setting, and data obtained in experimentally controlled situations. The review that follows will be restricted to modern accounts, specifically to those not suffering from the fundamental problems outlined in chapter 1. Optimally, these accounts should be classified along several dimensions:

Modality: Whether the description views the deficit as limited to production or as extended to comprehension as well; if the deficit is found in both modalities, whether it takes the same form.

Data Types: Whether the description focuses on agrammatic whole utterances or restricts itself to words or other linguistic types as produced or comprehended by agrammatics.

Focus: Whether the description concerns the structural properties of the agrammatic language or the processing mechanisms whose disruption is the cause of the functional deficit, or both.

Descriptive Framework: Whether a traditional structuralist grammar or a generative theory is used.

Goals: Clinical or theoretical.

It is not possible to present a coherent picture along so many dimensions. Therefore, the accounts reviewed below are presented only according to the modality on which they focus (although some are cross-modal generalizations) and according to whether they are devoted to the structural aspects of the agrammatic language or to (putatively disrupted) processes that underlie the impaired performance.

3.2   Agrammatic Speech Production

3.2.1   Processing Accounts
Since this part of the book focuses on structural aspects of agrammatic language, the discussion of processing issues will be relatively brief in terms of both comprehension and production. The review, though, is somewhat mixed: although it addresses claims concerning processes impaired and preserved in agrammatism, these can hardly be coherent unless at least some considerations of structure are taken into account. For this reason, at least some of the accounts to be reviewed are theories about both knowledge of language and its use in agrammatism; yet they all locate the deficit in a putative cognitive processing device or propose an account of how agrammatic speech is formed.

At a general level many proposals for the description of agrammatic speech exhibit striking similarities. That is, one finds accounts proposed fifty years apart that make very similar claims, varying only in degree of detail or in theoretical terminology. I will briefly review the main ones. Linguistically, they constitute two types: accounts that assume knowledge of the concept "sentence" and an ability on the part of agrammatic aphasics to use this knowledge, and accounts that do not.

Accounts assuming that agrammatic production indicates lack of awareness of the concept "sentence" have been offered by Luria (1970), Goodglass and Geschwind (1976), Saffran, Schwartz, and Marin (1980), and Caplan (1985).

(As we will see, Caplan's view differs slightly from the others'.) According to Saffran, Schwartz, and Marin, for instance, the agrammatic patient has a problem in "the translation of [semantic roles] into the sequence required by the linguistic code [that is, grammatical relations and whatever follows]" (p. 269). They claim, then, that agrammatic aphasics "are unable to map the underlying semantic structures into the N-V-N structure" (p. 270). This claim, coupled with the observation that agrammatic speech exhibits a preponderance of either infinitives (which are taken to be nominals) or -*ing* forms (which are taken to be gerunds) instead of finite verbs, leads these authors to conclude that "the agrammatic does not use the verb in a relational sense but rather to 'name' the action" (p. 278). The evidence for the last assumption (the nominal nature of verb forms in agrammatism) comes from Goodglass and Geschwind (1976), who conducted a comparative study of German- and English-speaking agrammatic patients and concluded that the verbs found in their speech are actually nominalizations. Observing an abundance of infinitives in the utterances of German-speaking patients, Goodglass and Geschwind take this evidence to resolve the question of whether agrammatics utter verbal or nominal forms, "since the German infinitive, unlike the English, has an inflectional ending. . . the agrammatic is not merely dropping the person and tense markers in English, but rather shifting to a nominalized form of the verb."

The obvious consequence of these claims is that even though the agrammatics have the ability to form an internal representation of the meaning of the proposition they wish to verbalize, they are unable to map the semantic representation onto syntactic form. It follows, then, that the patients either do not possess the concept "sentence" or can never realize it in their speech. This claim is extremely strong, since it assumes that agrammatics have lost most or even all of their syntax (or that they have no access to it). If all they have left is a naming ability, then it follows that they can use no syntactic processes in production (at least). Ignoring for the moment the susceptibility of this hypothesis to Occam's razor (since it is far from being parsimonious), empirical considerations alone are sufficient to reject it.

Two strong arguments can be put forth. The first comes from observations on agrammatic spontaneous speech. Saffran, Berndt, and Schwartz (1986), for instance, have recorded embeddings in agrammatic speech, such as "I'm gonna straighten up" and "I think I'll wear um dress." Though relatively rare in the patients' speech, these samples are far from being "automatized," frozen expressions, and they serve as an existence proof for preserved ability to implement recursive rules in language use, where the construct "sentence" is involved. This indicates awareness of this construct on the part of the patient.

The second, most detailed argument against the "naming" theory has been given by Lapointe (1985). I will briefly sketch its highlights. Lapointe shows, first of all, that Goodglass and Geschwind's argument is far from conclusive because the German infinitive is as ambiguous as its English counterpart with respect to grammatical analysis. That is, it may have either nominal or verbal identity. He then examines the properties of agrammatic utterances, showing that predictions made by the "naming" hypothesis are not borne out. Specifically, he shows that agrammatic utterances are always constrained by the argument structure of the verb and that patients produce sentences containing mixed morphological forms that demonstrate syntactic knowledge. That is, in a picture description task even severe agrammatics can produce sequences like *The boy is carr' in' the girl* and *The truck is pullin' the bus,* which suggests that the verbal forms they produce are transitive and not used as nominals. Also, the fact that the *-ing* morphology is occasionally omitted does not enable us to view the verbal forms produced as gerundive nominals.

Lapointe also cites evidence from other languages, where unambiguously finite verb forms have consistently been observed in agrammatic speech (Grodzinsky 1984a; Miceli et al. 1983). This evidence forces the tentative conclusion that whatever the deficit in agrammatic production is, knowledge and use of basic syntactic concepts such as "lexical category" and "sentence" are preserved. The "naming" hypothesis is not tenable. Nor is Caplan's (1985) weaker version, which assumes that agrammatics are aware of lexical categories but of nothing else. In particular, Caplan seems to deny the ability of agrammatics to construct phrasal categories. He is thus left with the claim that they do not serially produce sequences of nouns but instead utter N–V–N sequences that could constitute sentences but do not, because syntactic principles cannot relate the categories to one another. The difference between the "naming" hypothesis and Caplan's position, then, is minimal (although Caplan rejects the accounts of Luria and of Saffran, Schwartz, and Marin), for why would there be sequences of labeled syntactic categories if they could not make contact with syntax? Under Caplan's assumptions, knowledge of lexical categories would be of limited usefulness, if any: no grammatical processes may exploit this knowledge (because they are assumed to be lost), and the only processes that may utilize it are nonlinguistic (see below). Like Saffran, Schwartz, and Marin's theory, Caplan's predicts that an agrammatic utterance will not necessarily be well formed from the point of view of the argument structure of the verb it contains. This aspect of agrammatic language is well preserved, however, as Lapointe has convincingly demonstrated. In addition, Caplan's theory cannot account for the observed embeddings. (For further arguments against Caplan's analysis, see

corresponding to the two types of relations that structuralist linguists permitted among constituents: a *similarity* disorder, corresponding to the paradigmatic relation, and a *contiguity* disorder, corresponding to the syntagmatic relation. The former disturbance entails substitutions of lexical elements by words from the same category (a description that roughly fits the clinical description of paragrammatism in Wernicke's aphasia); the latter entails "loose" connections among words (supposedly accounting for the nonfluency in agrammatic aphasia). (A similar position is held by Goodglass and Mayer (1958), Luria (1970), and many others.)

Jakobson's account is formulated in structuralist terms. Arguments against this general approach have been amassed in the last thirty years and need not be repeated here. Suffice it to say that this theory lacks explanatory force and that as a description of agrammatism it is inadequate. The Regression Hypothesis has been tested empirically, although the putative negative results of this research will be questioned later. (See many of the papers in Caramazza and Zurif 1978a for conceptual and empirical evaluations of this very interesting hypothesis.) As for the similarity/contiguity account, it has two flaws. The "contiguity" disorder may be anything, for all practical purposes. There is nothing in the characterization of this disorder that specifies the omission of the closed-class vocabulary items and the retention of the rest. All it says is that connections among words will not be as tight as in normal speech. Clearly, this does not account for the basic facts. Under this description, for instance, agrammatism could consist in the omission of content words and the retention of the rest. Moreover, Jakobson's account predicts Broca's and Wernicke's aphasias to be in complementary distribution; yet, given that these aphasias are caused by physical agents that are presumably insensitive to linguistic distinctions, such a relation between the two diseases would be miraculous. It would mean that considerations of cognitive functioning determine the distribution of blood vessels in the brain. So, although Jakobson definitely deserves to be credited as a pioneer of the interaction between linguistics and neuropsychology, his specific theoretical proposals regarding agrammatism are inadequate.

For years afterward the topic was neglected, until in the 1970s the structural properties of language in agrammatism returned to the limelight and began to be subjected to fairly thorough investigation. Several accounts have been offered, making use of concepts borrowed from generative grammar. The first claims of this kind were actually made in the late 1950s but received little attention. Goodglass and Hunt (1958) used the theoretical framework proposed by Chomsky (1957) to account for the finding that English-speaking agrammatic patients omit fewer plural morphemes than possessive *s*'s even though the two morphemes sound alike. Following a suggestion by Morris Halle, they observed that, according to the theory of syntax Chomsky had proposed, constructions containing the possessive morpheme were derived by a transformation (*John's book* from *John has a book*), whereas constructions containing the plural morpheme were not. They characterized the speech pattern of agrammatic Broca's patients accordingly: transformationally derived *s*'s are omitted, whereas base-generated ones are not. In adopting this strategy, Goodglass and Hunt used a grammatical concept to distinguish impaired and preserved elements. What they failed to do, however, was to state a generalization. Had they proposed, say, that categories that change position as a result of a transformational operation were impaired, and the rest were left intact, then their account would have provided a testable hypothesis. But their account was formulated in an ad hoc fashion, to fit a single finding. As a result, no predictions followed, and no further experimentation was conducted to pursue the hypothesis, which was subsequently abandoned.

It was nearly twenty years later when Kean (1977) proposed the next linguistic characterization of agrammatism. Concerned to provide a linguistically coherent account of the omission patterns in the syndrome, she suggested distinguishing the omitted from the spared elements in speech by phonological means. Examining the existing partition between the two types of elements—the open- versus closed-class (content versus function) words—she argued that this commonly used distinction made no sense syntactically or morphologically, since neither group of elements formed a natural class at either of these levels of grammatical representation in modern linguistic theory. Hence, to characterize agrammatism as a syntactic or morphological disturbance, Kean claimed, is totally ad hoc. She instead proposed a natural distinction between the two groups of words that can be found at the *phonological* level of the grammar. She argued that although the lexical categories of the content words N, A, V do not cluster together morphologically, syntactically, or semantically, the contrast between the concepts "phonological word" and "clitic"—independently motivated phonological notions—correctly distinguishes the content words and the function words. The distinction follows quite naturally from a particular definition of word boundaries that the theory of generative phonology provides. Thus, the phonological level is the correct locus of a natural distinction between the impaired and preserved linguistic elements in agrammatism, resulting in the following linguistic description of agrammatism: "A Broca's aphasic tends to reduce the structure of a sentence to the minimal string of elements which can be lexically construed as phonological words in his language" (Kean 1977, 25).

Kean's proposals generated several reactions and intensified the linguistic discussion of agrammatism. Her phonological framework was challenged (Klosek

1979), and alternative formulations were proposed. Lapointe (1983) provides a formalism that attempts to capture the same range of data by a morphological generalization. Lapointe recasts Kean's analysis in morphological terms showing that, contrary to her claim, the phonological description of agrammatism is not unique and that a natural distinction between the (omitted) closed- and (spared) open-class items can also be found in morphology.

Lapointe is concerned to construct an alternative to the phonological description of agrammatism. If his arguments are correct, then at best his and Kean's accounts are extensionally equivalent. And, if one takes the view assumed here concerning deficit descriptions, this is not particularly enlightening. As descriptive statements, formal characterizations of language deficits do not have to be unique. They are in the business of providing non–ad hoc, adequate partitions of the data, and nothing else. Uniqueness of analysis is necessary just in case explanatory power is sought. Yet both Kean's and Lapointe's accounts offer only a descriptive generalization over data patterns, not an explanation. Indeed, both of these authors fail to draw theoretical conclusions from their descriptions of agrammatism (for a critique, see Grodzinsky 1985). Alternative formulations of the same pattern thus neither diminish nor strengthen the claims. From the present perspective, the difference between Kean's and Lapointe's accounts can be ignored.

Though these proposals are coherent and well motivated, there are empirical problems with both. One problem arises in connection with languages with morphological types that do not fit the English pattern. Consider inflected elements, for instance. Kean's description predicts that stems (what she calls "phonological words") will be retained in agrammatic speech, and inflections omitted. This raises the following questions: (1) What happens if the inflection changes the stem, without changing its status as a phonological word? That is, what happens in a case where inflection is an operation *internal* to the word, as in *take → took* or *make → made*? (2) What if the uninflected stem is not a word, a phenomenon unattested in English but well documented in many other languages?[2] Kean's proposals do not address these issues, because universally, there is no perfect overlap between stems and phonological words on the one hand, and inflections and clitics on the other. Consider *take,* for instance. Suppose an agrammatic patient would like to express its past tense. Will the patient omit anything, inflect correctly, or always stay with the present form? According to Kean's hypothesis, such expressions pose no special problems, because either form—present or past—is a phonological word. Production should remain intact, since both can be "construed as phonological words." Only when inflection manifests itself as the addition of a clitic morpheme—as in *rak-ed,* for example—is omission predicted. Below we will see that this prediction is incorrect, because omission is not the only type of error that agrammatic patients make.

The significance of this point is further emphasized when we consider languages with morphological properties that differ from those of English. This brings us to the second question, concerning words that lack a zero-inflection option. The relevant examples come from languages that have elements that inflect without a zero-option. There are two distinct cases. In one case, illustrated for example by certain elements in Russian and Italian, the uninflected element (stem) is a legal phonological sequence but not a phonological word. The second case is attested in Hebrew, where the uninflected element—the verbal root—does not even constitute a phonetically pronounceable string and a fortiori is not a phonological word. In both cases Kean's account again predicts that no problem would arise for agrammatic aphasics. Since the stem (or root) becomes a phonological word only when inflected, the inflection is contained within the phonological word. Thus, if agrammatic aphasics reduce their speech to phonological words, then no errors would be observed in these cases.

In Grodzinsky 1984a I address these issues by taking an extreme example and giving it a detailed treatment. I argue that since the phonological theory assumed by Kean is of limited generality, a description based on it cannot be considered universal. Specifically, the scope of the theory from which the distinction between phonological words and clitics is said to follow (the theory of Chomsky and Halle 1968) is limited to languages whose morphology resembles that of English. Yet languages with nonconcatenative morphology (McCarthy 1981)—most notably Semitic languages—cannot be described by this theory. Consequently, Kean's characterization cannot account for the agrammatic deficit in these languages.

Let us consider the formal properties of Kean's proposal in more detail. The linguistic elements that are crucially at issue are the so-called inflectional elements (such as *-ed, -ing, -s*) that are omitted from agrammatic speech in languages like English. The phonological theory that Kean assumes has an algorithm that annotates strings for word boundaries. The resulting representation distinguishes among different types of words by the "strength" of the boundaries that surround them. Phonological words are flanked by "thicker" boundaries than clitics. It is this distinction that Kean proposes to exploit for the description of omission patterns in agrammatism. She proposes that phonological words are spared and clitics omitted in agrammatic speech. This statement gives a linguistically motivated means for distinguishing between the two groups of words.

A crucial assumption for this account is that the relevant elements are continuous and that sequences of elements are linearly organized—in other words, that the retained phonological words lie next to the omitted clitics. This is because the process of segmentation (by word boundaries) operates on linearly ordered sequences. But this assumption is false in nonconcatenative languages. In these languages morphemes are not ordered sequentially but instead interwoven. The difference between the two language types is shown in (1). (1a) contains a schema for an English word, and (1b) a representation of a Semitic word. The English inflectional morphology follows the stem, whereas the Semitic inflection inheres in the vowel pattern that forms the skeleton into which the consonantal meaning-bearing "root" is *inserted*.

(1) a. STEM + CL ⟶ [#[#word#]inflection#]
         walk + ed ⟶ walk ed
     b. C_C_C + prefix-_V_V_V-suffix ⟶ prefixCVCVCsuffix
         k l x + hit-_a_ a_ 0-nu ⟶ hitkalaxnu

The symbols [# and #] in (1a) designate the word boundary that constitutes the criterion for omission, according to Kean. That is, only words flanked (by the algorithm proposed by Chomsky and Halle) with these symbols on both sides count as phonological words. Since inflections are flanked on one side only, they are clitics. As such, they are omitted. We now have a formal criterion for omission, provided by the boundary-assigning algorithm. Yet in (1b) no such boundary exists, because the annotation algorithm cannot work. As is obvious from (1), the phonology of such languages must be described by appealing to a formalism that contains different tiers, rather than bracketed sequences. Kean's account predicts that in this case no grammatical aberration will arise. A priori this appears unlikely, and in the next paragraph we will see that it is actually false. At this stage, then, Kean's generalization is suspect, since it seems inapplicable to any language with morphology that does not respect word boundaries the way English does.

The schema in (1) also suggests that the clinical description of agrammatism as "omission" of function words is suspect. If the Semitic inflection is omitted in agrammatism, then patients should either produce unpronounceable roots, sequences of consonants without vocalic skeletons (which would presumably be omitted), or omit every inflecting category, in which case they would be virtually mute. Both predictions are intuitively strange, and as expected they are both false. The patients can speak, and their omission pattern is constrained by lexical well-formedness criteria. That is, a part of a word cannot be omitted if the remainder would be ill formed lexically. Examples of spontaneous speech patterns in various languages are given in (2), taken from Goodglass 1976, Grodzinsky 1984a, Tsvetkova and Glozman 1978, Miceli et al. (1983), and Panse and Shimoyama (1955).

(2) a. *English*
         Uh, oh, I guess six month...my mother pass away.

     b. *Hebrew*
         tiylu   anaxnu ba'ali   ve'ani
         took-a-walk (3rd person pl., masc.+fem.) we   my-husband and I

         xamesh   yamim
         five (fem.) days (masc.)

     c. *Russian*
         grustnaja   malchik
         sad (fem.)   boy (masc.)

         stol stoyit,   vot, stol stoyat,   stoyit[3]
         table stands (sing.), lo,   table stand (pl.), stands

         rebionek prishl v shkolu...   shkole
         child   come to school (acc.) school (gen.–wrong)

     d. *Italian*
         Cappuceto   rossa   andava
         Little Ridinghood (masc.) Red (fem.) went

     e. *Japanese*
         inorimasu (correct: inorimasushita)[4]
         I-pray   I-prayed

Clearly, nonwords are not produced. Moreover, even in languages with "continuous morphology," if omission of an inflection would result in a nonword (for instance, s*toy* in (2c), *ross* in (2d), *inorima* in (2e)), the morpheme whose omission would cause the string to be ill formed is spared. The immediate conclusion is that word parts can be omitted only if zero-inflection is an option, contrary to Kean's prediction. Such is the English case: the singular form in the nominal system and the present tense form in the verbal system are both uninflected. Consequently, plurals, possessives, and verbal inflections are omitted in English agrammatic speech. But in languages such as Russian, Italian, and Hebrew, where omission of the nominal, adjectival, and verbal morphology would result in lexical ill-formedness, such elements are not omitted (although other closed-class items are). Rather, certain inflectional elements are *substituted* for others. In Hebrew this is due to the nonconcatenative nature of the morphology, and in the other languages it is due to the fact that in many instances there is no zero-inflection option. Thus, the questions raised at the beginning of this section have a clear answer: If omission would result in a nonword, then there is no omission; instead, the correct inflection is replaced by another inflectional option that the morphology permits. In Russian, for instance, the word *sumka* 'bag' has seven case inflections (*sumka, sumki, sumku,* and so on); the stem *sumk* is a nonword. Thus, Russian-speaking agrammatics err by producing words in the wrong case, yet each word is itself lexically well formed.

Kean's account is wrong, then, because it is based on one type of error—omission—whereas in reality both omissions and substitutions are observed. Since words are always well formed in agrammatic speech (barring phonemic paraphasias, which do appear, though rarely, in the speech of agrammatics), the linguistic description of agrammatism must refer to a level beyond the word. Indeed, the deviations from normal grammar observed in Russian, Italian, and Hebrew agrammatism arise when the wrong inflectional element is selected, resulting in violations of agreement, tense, aspect, and so on. Since these features appear at some syntactic level, the correct description of agrammatism must be syntactic.

Going back to the clinical literature, we find that at least one group of authors (Tissot, Mounin, and Lhermitte 1973) refer, though vaguely, to syntactic features as relevant to characterizing the agrammatic deficit. For these authors, one of the "defining traits" of the syndrome is the "lack of agreement." Yet they make no attempt to couch this observation within a theoretical framework, to yield a well-articulated descriptive generalization. In Grodzinsky 1984a I proposed one such account, which I will modify in the discussion that follows.

3.2.2.2   The Formal Characterization of Agrammatic Speech   In general, one could imagine two approaches to the linguistic description of language deficits. The first seeks to distinguish the linguistic elements whose use is impaired from those that are preserved. To this end, grammatical concepts are borrowed (from some theory) in order to partition the data correctly. In essence, all the accounts reviewed in the previous section adopt this approach. Goodglass and Hunt (1958), for example, say that agrammatics omit transformationally derived suffixes and retain the rest; Kean (1977) claims that they tend to reduce their speech to phonological words only. Generally, then, these accounts are of the form "Patient X does Y to Z," where X is a clinical type (Broca's aphasia, Wernicke's aphasia, etc.), Y is a behavioral type (proper use, omission, substitution, etc.), and Z is a grammatical type (lexical or phrasal category, phonological word, etc.). Grammatical concepts play a rather marginal role in such descriptions, for they merely pick out the elements that are treated pathologically by the patients. The precise nature of this treatment needs to be specified (by the *Y* variable in the formula). This is actually not surprising, because these accounts do not go beyond the observed behavior. So, although all of these proposals use grammatical distinctions in order to divide agrammatic speech into the omitted and retained elements and thus account for the observed speech patterns, none of them makes claims concerning the *grammatical representation* of these aberrant utterances. The second type of deficit description remedies this deficiency. Instead of simply distinguishing the impaired elements from the retained ones, this type of account answers the question, how could the language system be impaired so that it *represents* such strings as grammatical? In other words, instead of simply describing behaviors, such an account seeks out underlying mechanisms. In this case the task is to specify a change in the representational system—a change that characterizes the difference between normal and pathological language as attested in agrammatic speech.

This can be achieved in several ways. First, one could make a new, "aphasic" grammar, bearing no particular relation to normal grammar. If tailored carefully, such a grammar could fit the data from aphasia. Nevertheless, it would teach us nothing about normal linguistic systems. From our present perspective behavioral disturbances are interesting because they are encountered in previously normal individuals, and the theoretical statements we propose must reflect the change in the mechanisms that underlie their behavior. Yet if we construct a completely new grammar, we miss the main point. The goal of neuropsychological research—to learn about the normal from the pathological—cannot be achieved in this way. We must therefore take normal grammar as our point of departure and modify it when we encounter behavioral aberration. We will begin our descriptive effort by assuming that the impaired system is normal, unless otherwise demonstrated. Our null hypothesis, then, is that there is no impairment—we assume the *most minimal deficit possible*. This position is not universally accepted. Caplan and Futter (1986), for instance, propose the opposite. They begin their description with a minimal grammar—not one that is most similar to normal, but one that assumes that no knowledge is represented and that adds more assumptions as the data require. Yet doing that is like modifying a regular suit for an amputee by first tearing it apart and then reconstructing it, rather than by the more seemingly rational method of removing small parts (half a sleeve, say) piecemeal.

We can modify the grammar in either of two ways: by changing or dropping grammatical principles, or by modifying representations. Since the claims we wish to make are psychological (about the mechanism that underlies aberrant behavior), the following considerations must be taken into account. If we modify rules, we claim that the deficit arose from a strictly grammatical deficiency, not from the processor. But this need not be the case in principle. The loss may affect either the system of grammatical knowledge or the processor that implements it. Most importantly, we cannot know a priori what was disrupted. It is therefore best not to make a commitment on this point, at least at the outset. We can avoid having to make this commitment by modifying grammatical representations instead of rules. We can say then that the representations are abnormal, and that the abnormality may arise from either grammatical or processing deficiencies. That is, the representation may be abnormal either because knowledge has been lost or because a mechanism has been disrupted. Modifying a representation is therefore the most general form of a deficit description, and this is what I propose below.

The deficit analysis of agrammatic speech that I will propose focuses, first of all, on the inflectional morphology in agrammatic utterances. It takes the formalism provided by the current linguistic theory whose essentials are stated in Chomsky 1981 and modifies it to yield an adequate description of agrammatism. In order to account for cross-linguistic patterns, it begins with the assumption that in agrammatism certain features at the syntactic level that contains annotated surface structures—S-structure level—are underspecified. S-structure is the level at which constituents appear in their surface order in an annotated representation, where marking of transformational operations, definiteness, and the like appear. It is at this level that the lexical value of a category (N, V, A) and its inflectional properties (tense, agreement, and so on) are specified. S-structure is also the input for the phonological component that translates the annotated representation into phonological notation, called Phonological Form (PF).

I propose that in agrammatism the specific values of features like Agreement—person, gender, and number—are not given. This is achieved by deleting the values of these features from the representation. Now violations of agreement and related features are permitted. This is so because a representation is well formed just in case there is a match in agreement features between, say, the subject and the predicate; in the case of underspecified representations, features cannot be checked for matches or mismatches since feature values are deleted. As a result, any value (whether matching or not) may be chosen—any lexical element compatible with any value of a given feature may be selected—and the representation will still be well formed.

The features involved here are dominated by the INFL node, an abstract category that contains terminal nodes specifying all the inflectional features of predicates. INFL usually has the internal structure shown in (3).

(3)   INFL

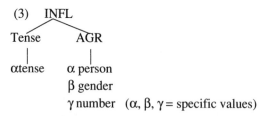

Tense   AGR
  | |
αtense   α person
            β gender
            γ number   (α, β, γ = specific values)

The formal description of these phenomena (which is a partial account of agrammatism) can now be stated as shown in (4).

(4) The value of features contained in INFL is deleted in agrammatism.

To illustrate with a hypothetical example from Hebrew, the abbreviated normal representation in (5a) will be replaced in the "agrammatic" grammar by the one in (5b), thus permitting Hebrew sentences like those in (5c–e), where in normal grammar (5c) is grammatical, and the others are not.

(5)a. [ha-yeled [KTB   INFL[+future, +3rd person +sing., +masc.]] sefer]
        the boy   write (root)   a book

   b. [ha-yeled [KTB INFL   [αtense, βperson, γgender] sefer]

   c. ha-yeled yiktob   sefer
      the-boy   will write a book (correct)

   d.*ha-yeled   kotebet   sefer
      the-boy   writing [feminine, present] a book

   e.*ha-yeled   katbu   sefer
      the-boy   wrote [past, plural]   a book

Thus, in addition to accepting every normally grammatical sentence, a representational system modified in this way will accept as grammatical certain sentences that the normal system rejects as ungrammatical.[5] The result is a language that is larger than normal.

The statement in (4) raises two questions. First, given the underspecification account that covers Hebrew, Italian, and Russian substitutions, why would agrammatism in languages like English manifest itself in *omissions*? That is, what role do considerations of lexical well-formedness play here, and is the English omission related to the fact that English words have a zero-inflection option? Second, what about the other elements that are involved in the agrammatic linguistic disorder, such as determiners, prepositions, and complementizers? How do these behave in languages whose morphologies differ from that of English, and how can the account be modified to accommodate these elements naturally?

To answer the first question, we must first examine the patterns of omission and substitution and their relation to the grammatical properties of the language at issue. There are two possibilities: (1) Agrammatism will always be manifested by omission in languages like English whose morphology permits it, and it will always be manifested by substitution in languages whose morphology does not always have a zero-inflection option. (2) Agrammatism will be manifested by omission when the lexical item in question permits, otherwise by substitution. In short, the question is whether agrammatics' behavior in the production of inflected elements is tied to the properties of the word they happen to utter or to the language they speak. Possibility 1 would mean that English-speaking agrammatics would always omit and that Russian-speaking agrammatics would always substitute. It would also mean that the structural account must be stated parametrically, with the parameter(s) relating to the morphology of the language spoken. Possibility 2 would mean that what determines the production pattern is a very local consideration: if a word is well formed without inflection, it would appear; otherwise, it would take some inflectional form, though not necessarily the correct one. In this case the language type itself is immaterial.

The little existing evidence on this issue points toward the second possibility. That is, the error pattern appears to be item-bound. Take Russian, for instance. In this language inflected elements tend to be substituted. The crucial test that will decide between the two possibilities is provided by Russian words that have a zero-inflection option. If in spite of the zero-inflection option agrammatic speakers substitute, then the language is the relevant distinctive variable. If, however, they omit inflections in such items rather than substituting one for another, then the error pattern is item-bound. Tsvetkova and Glozman (1978) provide some relevant cases. The Russian word *snjeg* 'snow' is uninflected in the nominative case and takes suffixes (*snjega, snjegu, snjego*, and so forth) in the other cases. Possibility 1 would predict substitution, and possibility 2 omission. The data show omission in this case. The flip side of this test comes from English, where elements are generally omitted. Here, if we found a word that does not have a zero-inflection option, possibility 2 would predict substitution under the assumption that such a word has no single, "basic" form. Such elements may be words with "strong," irregular inflection, such as those in (6).

(6) Nouns: foot, goose, mouse, louse, etc.
     Verbs: go, seek, bring, sing, etc.

I am aware of no data bearing on this issue from English, and future empirical work is necessary. Nevertheless, the Russian (and some Italian) data suggest that the production pattern is item-bound and not language-bound (contrary to the claims in Grodzinsky 1984a). This being the case, we can say that lexical well-formedness considerations are operative in agrammatism. What is violated are syntactic well-formedness conditions. We must therefore reduce the grammar so that it will permit the violations that are observed. As noted earlier, however, we may modify only representations, not rules of grammar. The statement in (4) has precisely the desired properties and consequences: it underspecifies features at some syntactic level but keeps grammatical rules, and particularly rules of word formation, intact. To meet conditions on lexical well-formedness, then, a word *must* be inflected if it does not have a zero-form; since the specification of inflectional dimensions is incomplete, the agrammatic speaker must resort to guessing, which sometimes results in violations of agreement, tense, and aspect.[6] On the other hand, if a word is well formed without inflecting, there would be no inflection if the inflectional dimensions are underspecified, because inflection would not be forced by conditions on lexical well-formedness. We thus have a grammatical system from which the cross-linguistic (actually, cross-lexical) pattern of error follows. In particular, no "default mechanism" such as the one assumed in Grodzinsky 1984a needs to be stipulated.[7] Underspecification makes the default automatic. If the material on the left branch of a representation like those in (7) need not combine with the material on the right branch to form a word, then omission follows, as in (7a). However, if the left branch does not contain a well-formed word, it will need to combine with some inflectional element to form a word; for want of specification, it will pick anything compatible with the representation, and substitution will follow, as in (7b).

(7)   a.

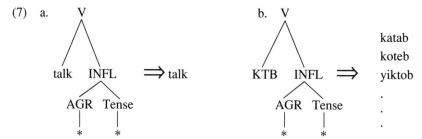

In sum, (4) makes the grammar more permissive than it normally is: a grammatical system restricted by (4) permits the normal language and more. Specifically, it predicts that agrammatic aphasics will produce sentences that contain agreement violations, which is indeed the case. It follows that the agrammatic language is *larger* in size than the normal language, because the agrammatic grammar generates all the normal language and more. This property has implications that I discuss in chapter 6.

So far I have concentrated on inflected words. Obviously, however, these are not the only problematic items in agrammatism. The clinical description states that prepositions, determiners, auxiliaries, and complementizers (the so-called free-standing function words) are omitted in agrammatic speech. As far as is known, these tend to be omitted in every language in which they appear. Can the account in (4) be extended to include them, as well?

To begin with, let us exclude prepositions from the remaining group. We will deal with them separately, for reasons I will give later. We are then left with grammatical, as opposed to lexical, formatives (the lexical categories). But note that INFL, the crux of the statement in (4) regarding inflected elements, is also not a lexical category. This immediately suggests that the notion "nonlexical" is relevant for the description of agrammatism. (For a recent discussion of the contrast between lexical and nonlexical (or functional) categories, see Speas 1986.) Specifically, if we say that nonlexical elements are underspecified at S-structure, we capture the data. To do this, however, we need a clear definition of the notion "lexical." I will consider two alternatives, formulated in accordance with Chomsky's (1981, 1986b) definitions of lexical categories, and examine their consequences. The restriction on agrammatic representations is now as formulated in (8).

(8) In agrammatism, nonlexical terminals are deleted from S-structure representation.

Definition
A terminal element is lexical iff:
Definition 1: It is dominated by a category defined by the features $[\pm N, \pm V]$.
Definition 2: It contains lexical material at a given level.

Several points deserve comment here. First, the restriction is on *terminal elements* that are "leaves" of the tree, that is, elements that dominate nothing. Second, consider the consequences of the restriction under each definition of "lexical." Under definition 1, nonlexical elements are determiners, complementizers, adverbs, inflection, auxiliaries, and case markers.[8] Under definition 2, nonlexical elements are determiners, inflection, auxiliaries, and case markers, as well as the empty categories trace and PRO and their associated indices. I am aware of no data that distinguish between the two definitions, although they make different predictions. In addition, there are other potential considerations that may decide the issue. We may thus leave the notion "lexical" in (8) ambiguous until we have the relevant data.

I have shown how the proposal in (8) accounts for the inflectional errors made by agrammatics. However, I have so far said nothing about derivational morphology. Indeed, the state of affairs on this front is far from clear. To my knowledge, there is no systematic study of derivational errors in agrammatism. It should be noted, however, that according to (8) no derivational errors should ever occur. Theories of morphology differ with respect to the level at which morphological processes take place. Yet in all the theories I am aware of, derivational morphemes are not under the restriction stated in (8). Derivational morphemes are mostly dominated by a lexical category and are never repre-sented by empty categories. Thus, they satisfy either definition of "lexical." Hence, they are always lexical and are predicted to be intact.[9]

It now remains to account for the omission of prepositions in agrammatism. Can this be accomplished by extending the account in (8), or is an additional statement necessary? As stated, the characterization in (8) cannot be modified to cover prepositions, because the crucial notion in (8) is "lexical," distinguish-ing grammatical formatives from the categories N, V, A, P. Since according to the proposed account all the lexical categories cluster together, we are barred from extending it to prepositions in a non–ad hoc fashion. This formal argument favoring the distinction between grammatical formatives and prepositions receives further empirical support, which saves it from being ad hoc. This support comes from findings that point toward selective impairment within the prepositions. Friederici and her colleagues have shown that some prepositions are omitted and others are retained (Friederici 1982; Friederici, Schonle, and Garrett 1982; Friederici 1985).

There are several hypotheses concerning the precise distinction between the two groups. Everyone agrees that the lexical identity of the preposition is irrelevant for the characterization; rather, distributional properties determine the pattern of impairment and sparing. The debate centers around the property that makes the distinction. Friederici and her colleagues maintain that the distinction is "lexical" versus "semantic"—that lexically determined (strictly subcatego-rized) prepositions are omitted and semantically determined ones are spared. This distinction is insufficient, as I have shown (Grodzinsky 1984a, 1988), because the contrast "lexical" versus "semantic" does not cover all the cases and is not based on a clear, theoretically motivated distinction. Another proposal has been made by Rizzi (1985), who claims that thematic properties of categories determine their fate. On his account, elements assigning theta-roles are pre-served, and the rest are impaired. The theory he follows (GB Theory) specifies which elements assign a theta-role and which do not. As I have shown (Grodzinsky 1984a, 1988), this account is also inadequate, because it ties the deficit to specific words, which seems to give wrong predictions here. Specifically, it predicts that the only preposition to be omitted in English is *of,* since (according to GB

Theory) *of* is the only English preposition that never assigns a theta-role. As alternatives, I have proposed two similar accounts of the distinction. Both make the claim that the omitted and spared prepositions differ configurationally. In Grodzinsky 1984a I have proposed that prepositions contained in a PP that is a daughter of S are the only ones retained. On this account, based on Friederici's data, particles (as in *called John up*) are not prepositions but are reanalyzed as part of the verb; hence, they are retained. Temporal and locative prepositions and the passive *by* are also retained. The account predicts that subcategorized prepositions, as in *believe in God,* will be omitted, since the phrases that contain them are daughters of VP, not of S (that is, [PP,VP]). Therefore, prepositions that are heads of daughters of VP are omitted whereas reanalyzed particles and heads of adjuncts are preserved, which leads to the above formulation. In Grodzinsky 1988 I have modified this account slightly. Based on further experimental evidence, I claim in that work that the notion "government," taken from GB Theory, provides the correct distinction. Specifically, prepositions that are governed (that is, subcategorized prepositions, heads of PPs in ditransitive verbs) are omitted, and the rest are preserved. Thus, the correct account of the selective deficit with respect to prepositions in agrammatism is as shown in (9).

(9)   In agrammatism, governed prepositions are deleted; all others are retained.

This characterization apparently accounts for the deficit in both the production and the comprehension of prepositions. Combining the account for grammatical formatives with the account for prepositions, the universal characterization of the grammatical representations for agrammatic speech production patterns is as shown in (10).

(10) At S-structure the representation of agrammatic speech differs from the representation of normal speech in the following respects:
   a.   Nonlexical terminals are deleted.
   b.   Governed prepositions are deleted.

Thus, an impoverished representation in the above sense is the grammatical characterization of agrammatic production.

     As pointed out to me by Doug Saddy, this proposal fails to account for one important piece of data. Zurif and Caramazza (1976) tested patients' ability to construct sentences from written fragments. Among other things, they found a contrast in performance with respect to different uses of the preposition *to.* Patients did well when to functioned as a dative preposition (as in *John gave the book to Mary*) but performed poorly when it was infinitival (as in *John wanted to leave*). Assuming that this task somehow reflects production, this performance pattern is not predicted by the account in (10), because *to* is governed in both cases and therefore should yield poor performance in both. We now have compelling evidence in support of the claim that agrammatism is indeed a grammatical problem: different languages exhibit different error patterns that are explained by referring to different grammatical factors.

The proposed description has several important implications. First, it makes no claim regarding the source of the impairment in agrammatism—whether it arises from a disrupted language processor or from a deficient knowledge of grammar. All it defines is the notion of "grammaticality" in agrammatism (for production), a notion more permissive than normal. Second, the fact that prepositions and other elements are accounted for separately raises the possibility that the source of the impairment in each case is different. Third, the definition of the notion "lexical" is ambiguous, pending further investigation. We will see that this definition is relevant to the so-called parallelism issue: whether or not the production deficit parallels the comprehension deficit in agrammatism will crucially depend on this definition. Fourth, the account differs descriptively from previous ones (Kean 1977; Lapointe 1983) in four respects: (1) Rather than focusing on a morphophonological level, it shifts the descriptive burden to the syntax, thus deriving both the classical omission pattern and cross-linguistic variation in agrammatic production. (2) It contends that the generalization over inflectional elements and prepositions is spurious and that they actually require two separate statements. (3) It accounts for aberrant speech patterns by modifying the grammar, not just by using grammatical distinctions. (4) The phonological account for prepositions is based on the false assumption that these elements are impaired regardless of their syntactic context. By contrast, the present characterization accounts for the differential impairment patterns observed for members of this category.

3.3 Agrammatic Comprehension

Among all the selective cognitive deficits known today, the comprehension deficit in agrammatic aphasia seems to me the most interesting and relevant to theoretical issues. Yet despite early observations of a comprehension deficit accompanying the typical agrammatic production deficit, the literature records no systematic discussion on this topic prior to the early 1970s.[10] At that time Zurif and his colleagues began a comprehensive survey of the comprehension abilities of agrammatic patients (see, among others, Zurif, Caramazza, and Meyerson 1972; Zurif et al. 1974; Zurif and Caramazza 1976; Caramazza and Zurif 1976), and about a decade later a body of data and several theoretical accounts were already available. In this section I will review these accounts and propose an alternative. As in the discussion of speech production, I will distinguish between accounts that focus on the processing abilities of agrammatic patients and characterizations of their grammatical representations.

It has been widely known for some time that the traditional descriptions of agrammatism in Broca's aphasia were inaccurate. These amount to the statement that although Broca's patients' comprehension is almost unimpaired, grammatical formatives are invariably missing from their speech (Goldstein 1948; Goodglass and Kaplan 1972). In the first part of this chapter I argued against the traditional description of agrammatic speech production patterns. Yet there I discussed data that have been available for decades and offered a new generalization over well-known error patterns. In the domain of comprehension, by contrast, the first critique of the traditional description is motivated by relatively new data. The clinicians, using bedside methods to assess the comprehension of aphasic patients, formulated their characterizations on the basis of informal conversations rather than controlled experiments. Zurif and his colleagues challenged this view, pointing out that the comprehension limitation in agrammatic aphasia was wider in scope than had previously been supposed, and attempting to provide a model-based account of this limitation. As a result, interest in this limitation grew, and in the past decade many controlled experiments have attempted to assess the comprehension abilities of aphasics via the use of sound methods.

Once the agrammatic group of patients was shown to have some comprehension problems in the syntactic domain (see Caramazza and Zurif 1976; Zurif and Caramazza 1976; Schwartz, Saffran, and Marin 1980; Grodzinsky 1986a), a debate began about its exact nature that has continued ever since. Testimony to the intensity and broadness of this debate is the fact that the only point on which most investigators seem to agree is that the deficit goes beyond production and that all other modalities are involved to some degree. (Even this is true only if we set aside some exceptional cases. See Miceli et al. 1983; Kolk and van Grunsven 1985a.) Very little else is agreed upon. It is debatable, for example, whether the deficit in comprehension parallels the deficit in production; there are conflicting views about the fate of several grammatical formatives; and—most important in the present context—many investigators question the presence of a syntactic impairment.

Yet despite the disagreement, the study of the comprehension abilities of agrammatic aphasics has by and large focused on syntactic issues. From the first studies on agrammatic comprehension it seemed that the disturbance in this syndrome was somehow related to syntax. The crucial question concerned the exact relevance of syntax to the agrammatic impairment, and since the theoretical interpretation of the small body of data has been difficult, the nature of the agrammatic comprehension limitation is still undetermined. Indeed, virtually every logically possible position is represented in the literature: some have suggested that agrammatic aphasics have lost their syntax completely (Caramazza and Zurif 1976; Berndt and Caramazza 1980; Caplan and Futter 1986); it has also been claimed that the syntactic loss is partial (Grodzinsky 1984b; 1986a); and others have argued that in fact there is no syntactic impairment in agrammatic aphasia (Linebarger, Schwartz, and Saffran 1983; Schwartz et al. 1987). Note that the debate has very little direct theoretical import; in effect, the argument concerns the proper *description* of the impairment. This confusing situation is not surprising, however. It seems to typify areas of research where the empirical basis is shaky and impoverished. To begin our run through this maze, I will review past findings and past processing and grammatical deficit accounts. Then I will propose an alternative.

3.3.1 Processing Accounts

For present purposes, our main interest in language-processing accounts of agrammatism lies in the grammatical abilities of agrammatic patients in timed comprehension and in comprehension-related tasks. Since the relevance of this research area to the claims made in this book is limited, I will review it only briefly.

The most important single claim concerning language processing in agrammatism is due to Bradley, Garrett, and Zurif (1980) Attempting to capitalize on the old distinction between the closed- and open-class vocabulary groups, they began with two observations: (1) Closed- but not open-class words are omitted in agrammatism. (2) In speech errors (see Garrett 1975), open- but not closed-class items are subject to substitution errors. These observations led them to believe that there might be a parallel comprehension deficit to this production pattern. Bradley (1978) argued that for normal listeners, access to the members of the open class is frequency sensitive, whereas access to the closed class is insensitive to frequency; that is, the time it takes to retrieve a closed-class item is not a function of that item's frequency of occurrence in the language. She then claimed that because of the important role of closed-class items in constructing the phrasal analysis of an input string, access to these elements should not be influenced by their frequency in order to parse the string as quickly as possible. Later Bradley, Garrett, and Zurif tested agrammatic aphasics on a task similar to the one Bradley had used with normals. They made the surprising discovery that in agrammatism, access to the closed class is sensitive to word frequency just like access to the open class. This led them to hypothesize that the lexicon is normally partitioned into frequency-sensitive and frequency-insensitive "bins." In the former, all the words in the language are stored; in the latter, just the closed-class words. In the normal process of comprehension, they claimed there may be competition between the two access routes when a closed-class item is accessed, a competition that the frequency-insensitive route always wins. In agrammatism, however, this route is disrupted, thus accounting for the appearance of frequency sensitivity in agrammatic patients. Figure 3.2 illustrates this proposal.

The theory of "double representation" of closed-class words became quite popular, yet it very soon came under attack. Interestingly, all the attacks were made on empirical grounds, and none stemmed from conceptual or theoretical considerations. Thus, several attempts failed to replicate Bradley, Garrett, and Zurif's results (Gordon and Caramazza 1982; Segui et al. 1982, among others), and arguments were advanced concerning the materials used in the experiments (Gordon and Caramazza 1983). It seems to me, however, that Bradley, Garrett, and Zurif's model is susceptible to other types of criticism as well. Specifically, its conceptual motivation is functional, yet the details are never given: the authors argue that the closed-class access route is frequency neutral so that a phrasal analysis can be assigned rapidly, yet they offer no details of how this class participates in parsing. In fact, given that the closed-/open-class distinction is syntactically incoherent (as Kean (1977) argues quite convincingly), one would be inclined to suspect that as a group, the closed-class items do not participate in syntactic parsing at all, because there is no single syntactic generalization that subsumes them all.

Apart from this one, few processing accounts of agrammatic comprehension have been proposed.[11] Notable among these is the account offered by Berndt and Caramazza (1980). These authors claim, with little evidence, that the agrammatic comprehension limitation is due to a parsing problem. Yet this claim is quite vague. No specific parsing model is cited, no empirical work pertinent to

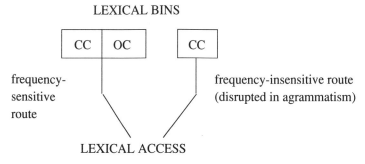

Figure 3.2

the claim is discussed in detail, and the claim itself is too general. As a result, little can be made of it.

3.3.2   Structural Accounts of Agrammatic Comprehension

Caramazza and Zurif (1976) were the first to propose an account of agrammatic comprehension that made an explicit claim about syntactic abilities in the syndrome. In a comprehension experiment they conducted, they reported the following results. First, they found that agrammatic patients were good at interpreting semantically "nonreversible" sentences, that is, sentences like (11a) where inferences can be made over lexical content to aid interpretation. But on semantically "reversible" sentences of a particular syntactic type like (11b), where full syntactic analysis is mandatory for interpretation, these patients performed poorly—in fact, at chance levels—indicating that they guessed at the correct answer.

(11) a. The ball that the boy is kicking is red.
     b. The girl that the boy is pushing is blond.

For (11b), the critical condition, the response sheet contained four possible answers: (a) a picture corresponding to the content of the sentence—the match (a boy and a girl); (b) a thematic foil, depicting reversal of theta-roles—the mismatch (a girl pushing a boy); (c) a distractor where the predicate adjective was changed (*blond* replaced by *black*); (d) a distractor where the verb in the relative clause was changed (*push* replaced by *kick*). The patients never chose the lexical distractors (c) and (d); thus, chance performance here means guessing between the match (a) and the mismatch (b). The response sheet given for (11a) is less clear. Was the mismatch just a lexical distractor, or one containing a ball kicking a boy—a nonsense situation to which real-life heuristics cannot be applied? The text does not reveal what was actually done, but no possibility lends itself to a straightforward interpretation. Indeed, as argued in Grodzinsky and Marek (1988), this part of the experiment was done incorrectly.

Performance levels in such experiments are measured by giving the subject 10–20 sentences in each condition, so that normal performance can be demonstrated, as distinct from guessing behavior or consistent misinterpretation. The task in this experiment was sentence-picture matching, where for every stimulus sentence there was a correct choice and several syntactic and semantic foils.

Caramazza and Zurif, however, gave this finding a radical interpretation: they took it to indicate that the patients "are unable to use syntactic-like algorithmic processes" (p. 581). All the patients could do, according to these authors, was to infer theta-roles from the semantics of words contained in each sentence, which meant that "they have retained the capacity to use heuristic procedures to assign a semantic interpretation to, at best, an incompletely represented syntactic organization" (p. 579). This is the reason for the discrepancy between their performance on reversible sentences and their performance on nonreversible sentences (whose syntactic analyses were kept constant).

This account makes two claims: (1) that syntactic processes in the comprehension device of agrammatic aphasics are inoperative, and (2) that aphasics can compensate for this disability by using heuristic strategies. These claims, as well as the data that motivated them, have been called into question. To take the second one first: It has been argued (Grodzinsky and Marek 1988) that the design of the experiment was flawed and that as a result the only interpretable finding concerned the reversible relatives like (11b). The argument turns on the methodology Caramazza and Zurif used in this study, which does not warrant claims about the use of semantic heuristics as alternative comprehension strategies that can bypass the aphasic impairment. The sentence-picture matching task cannot be used in the same way for the nonreversible as for the reversible sentences. In short, foils for sentences like (11a), depicting balls kicking boys, are either difficult to create or so bizarre that the patients simply ignore them. Moreover, they certainly do not lead the patients to invoke real-world heuristics, because they describe an imaginary situation in which such heuristics cannot work. Therefore, the sentence-picture matching task as devised by Caramazza and Zurif cannot test the use of heuristics. It follows that their claim that agrammatic patients use heuristics to compensate for their syntactic deficiency receives no support from this study, although in and of itself it seems quite plausible.

There are reasons to believe that the first claim made by Caramazza and Zurif's account—about asyntactic comprehension—is also flawed. Their interpretation of the finding is far too radical. An inability to use syntax may be consistent with the finding (chance-level performance on reversible relatives), yet from the examination of one syntactic construction, no matter how complex, one can hardly conclude that no syntax is available. In fact, this conclusion is acceptable only under the conception that knowledge of language is an undifferentiated (monadic) relation. On this view (discussed in chapter 1), if one finds a phenomenon relevant to one aspect of language, it must be relevant to all the other aspects to the same degree. In the present context, impaired performance on a single condition would thus count as evidence for a deficit cutting across all linguistic abilities. It seems, however, that the arguments against this conception of language are convincing, thus rendering the claim concerning total loss of syntactic abilities unmotivated; moreover, data from experiments that were conducted later clearly suggest that the impairment does not encompass all aspects of syntactic ability in these patients.

Caramazza and Zurif are not the only ones to have claimed that agrammatics have asyntactic comprehension. Caplan and Futter (1986) make a similar proposal, yet in a much more detailed fashion. They attempt to account for the performance of an agrammatic patient on a wide variety of syntactic constructions. The performance they observed was varied: sometimes the patient performed correctly, and sometimes she did not. To account for these findings, Caplan and Futter propose to assume that agrammatic aphasics retain only the ability to identify the syntactic category of a word. All other grammatical abilities are lost. As a consequence, agrammatic aphasics cannot analyze sentences syntactically, and they are reduced to relying on strategies. Caplan and Futter then propose some such strategies, attempting to derive the patient's performance from these.

In Grodzinsky 1986a,b I offered a critique of this proposal that made the following points. First, Caplan and Futter's proposal is descriptively inadequate. That is, application of the strategies they suggest would give results different from those actually observed. The linear strategy they assume is shown in (12).

(12) Assign the theta-roles of agent, theme, and goal to N_1, N_2, and N_3 in structures of the form $N_1-V-N_2-N_3$, where N_1 does not already bear a theta-role. (p. 128)

This statement is rather vague. The strategy is invoked as a default; that is, it is to be used when NPs have not been previously associated with theta-roles. Left unspecified, though, are the structures to which, and the manner by which, those previously associated roles are assigned. But even if taken literally, this strategy makes the wrong predictions: it associates the first noun with the role of agent, which predicts systematic inversion of theta-roles (agent for patient and vice versa) in constructions like passive and object-cleft sentences. since these are N–V–N structures (for instance, *The boy is pushed by the girl, It is the boy who the girl pushed*), the first N should be the agent, and the second the theme. The account thus predicts a performance level that is below chance, yet the patient studied by Caplan and Futter performed at chance levels on these syntactic types.

Second, there is a methodological flaw in Caplan and Futter's proposal, regarding the null hypothesis in the description of cognitive deficits. As noted in the previous section, I believe that the description of cognitive deficits is important because it may provide new insights into the structure of normal psychological mechanisms. Precisely for this reason, these deficits must always be described by comparison to what is taken to be the normal structure. After all, our object of inquiry is people who were mature, normal individuals until they were hit by cerebral disease that impaired their language skills. The null hypothesis, then, is that the mechanism in question is fully intact, unless there is evidence to the contrary. Only a demonstrated loss would lead us to hypothesize a disrupted piece of machinery in these patients' cognitive systems. On this view, then, one assumes minimal disruption to the patient's linguistic mechanisms. Any other description may be able to capture the patient's performance, but not in ways that may ever have any theoretical relevance. Caplan and Futter are concerned only with describing the patient's performance. They assume that she has no syntax—the most radical assumption—and then equip her with various strategies. Their account is not only unparsimonious but also formulated in such a way that connections between it and psychological theory are almost impossible.

On the other side of the debate we find Linebarger, Saffran, and Schwartz. In a series of papers they have argued that there is no syntactic deficit in agrammatism and that the aberrant performance can be attributed to the failure of other cognitive systems. Schwartz, Saffran, and Marin (1980), replicating findings by Goodglass (1968), report that on the comprehension of reversible passives agrammatic patients performed at chance levels. They argue that the problem is actually caused by a "mapping" deficit, in which the patient cannot map syntactic positions onto semantic roles. In a later experiment (Linebarger, Schwartz, and Saffran 1983) they found that patients who failed a standard comprehension test (containing reversible passives and relatives like those in (11)) were surprisingly successful at detecting ungrammaticality in a wide assortment of sentential types. This finding, they believed, confirmed their earlier claims that syntactic knowledge and processes are intact in agrammatism and that the problem lies in higher, syntacticosemantic mapping. We will see that this position, too, is tenable only under an undifferentiated view of language knowledge, according to which impairment to some aspect of syntax indicates that the whole syntactic knowledge base is gone.

Looking at the findings of Linebarger, Saffran, and Schwartz coupled with findings from other laboratories (see Ansell and Flowers 1982; Caplan and Futter 1986; Grodzinsky 1984b; Grodzinsky et al. 1988; Grodzinsky and Pierce 1987), we notice an interesting comprehension contrast. On reversible passives (13a), the patients perform at chance levels, but on actives (13b), their performance is above chance—indeed, it is virtually normal.

(13) a.   The boy was pushed by the girl.
     b.   The girl pushed the boy.

This contrast suggests immediately that a simple version of the "mapping" hypothesis is untenable. Under this hypothesis, there should be no performance difference among syntactic constructions in agrammatism, because syntactic structure is not a variable that interacts with the patient's deficiency. The claim is that patients cannot associate constituents with semantic roles and that this handicap is independent of any particular syntactic configuration. Syntax, according to the "mapping" hypothesis, is a single, unanalyzed variable. Proponents of this hypothesis thus ignore the contrast in agrammatic comprehension of structures such as (13a) and (13b), which suggests that for them, no distinctions among syntactic types are relevant. Still, even if they hold such a view, the contrast in (13) is unexpected from the standpoint of their own hypothesis. Also, the contrast reported by Linebarger, Schwartz, and Saffran (1983) between the good performance that patients exhibited on certain syntactic constructions and their poor performance on others not only remains a mystery but in fact goes against the position that the authors themselves articulate.[12] An attempt to restate the hypothesis must somehow incorporate a classification of constructions. This is what Schwartz et al. (1987) set out to do. Examining the successes and failures of agrammatic patients in a judgment task, they identify a syntacticosemantic mapping failure, concluding that agrammatic performance is determined by complexity considerations of a particular type. On their view, complexity should be measured relative to the "thematic transparency" of a construction, that is, with respect to how direct the assignment of theta-roles is. Thus, a structure containing an NP in a nonthematic position—a position that receives a theta-role not directly from an assigner but rather through its link to a mediating trace derived from transformational movement—is more complex and hence predicted to yield poorer performance than a structure in which all NPs are in thematic positions. So, although acknowledging the partial nature of the deficit, they maintain that the correct account is not syntactic. Yet the distinction they make between "hard" (complex) and "easy" (simple) constructions is in fact syntactic. Indirect versus direct theta-role assignment is a consequence of whether or not a transformational operation has occurred, resulting in a representation that contains a trace linked to an antecedent NP that receives a theta-role through the link. This syntactic distinction in fact makes up the core of the account proposed in Grodzinsky 1986a and refined in section 3.3.4. However, it is important to note that the proposal made by Schwartz et al., even if recast syntactically, is imprecise because it distinguishes between types of syntactic constructions but does not accurately predict the level of performance. As I will argue, "hard" and "easy" are unsatisfactory descriptive terms.

From the above data, it should be apparent that agrammatic comprehension is determined, at least in part, by variables that are tied to grammatical structure. The first notion that comes to mind is a partial syntactic deficit, which would be sensitive to construction type. On this view, there may be some constructions that do not cause problems to agrammatic patients, and some that do. This position is intermediate between the one claiming that agrammatic patients have lost their syntax and the one claiming that syntax in agrammatism is intact. We will see that in addition to being the only position compatible with most of the data, this account opens the way for imposing interesting constraints on theories of language structure and processing.

3.3.3 On Interpreting Data

Since at least some of the objections raised above are concerned with the proper interpretation of experimental findings and the nature of theoretical claims that are based on empirical observation, it is advisable to digress briefly on experimental issues. In this digression I will discuss what I see as the main variables involved in tasks related to language comprehension, and what interpretations of findings should take into account. In general, I will develop a simple theory of mapping, in the spirit of the theory of cognitive compiling developed by Hamburger and Crain (1984). These authors examine in detail the steps involved in carrying out one type of comprehension task and use this analysis to motivate a criticism of certain interpretations of children's linguistic knowledge. They point out that such a task minimally consists of grammatical analysis, planning, and execution of the plan. Each of these steps requires cognitive resources and capacities, the lack of which may give rise to errors in performance. They show that past claims concerning children's knowledge of grammar are at least dubious, and at most false, because they ignore these factors and ascribe every performance failure to a lack of linguistic knowledge. My attempt will be similar, though less ambitious. I will list some of the steps that are mandatory for carrying out a given task, in order to find loci of potential failure. First, however, we should consider several factors relevant to language comprehension in any experimental setting, namely, tasks, syntactic construction, and solution spaces.

The action a subject is requested to perform in an experiment is called the task. In the neuropsychology of language, the task most commonly used for testing the interpretive abilities of brain-damaged patients is *sentence-picture matching*. In this paradigm subjects hear (or read) a sentence, and then they are confronted with several line drawings, only one of which depicts a scene that matches the stimulus sentence. The dependent variable here is error rate, since performance on this task is usually not timed. However, many other tasks are also used in the study of language deficits. One of these is the *grammaticality judgment* task, in which subjects are presented (auditorily or visually) with a string of words and are asked to judge whether it constitutes a well-formed sentence in their language. On a view that takes language to be an unanalyzed entity, the kind of task used to probe linguistic ability is immaterial, because probing one linguistic variable is tantamount to examining the whole language. Yet if language is analyzable, and particularly if one can imagine linguistic deficits that are selective from a grammatical point of view, then the nature of the task used in experimentation becomes very important. Carrying out a given task may require resources of one type, which happen to be intact for some patient, whereas carrying out another task may crucially depend on a function that is impaired for that patient. As a consequence, any interpretation of a finding must incorporate a task analysis, whether explicit or implicit. The mapping from the stimulus up to the response has to be spelled out for a coherent interpretation to be given. For example, consider the task of giving a grammaticality judgment for a sentence like (14a), and compare it with the task of comprehending (14a)'s grammatical counterpart, (14b).

(14) a. *The boy is seen of the girl.
     b. The boy is seen by the girl.

To judge (14a) ungrammatical, one must know that *of* cannot appear in this context. Yet to interpret (14b) correctly, one must know the syntactic structure of the sentence and the correct thematic assignment. It is conceivable that there exist patients with an impairment that allows them to carry out one task successfully but causes them to fail on the other. In fact, at least one such finding has been reported concerning different types of passive constructions (Grodzinsky 1988). The choice of experimental task, then, is an extremely important factor in interpretation.

Other factors are no less important, however. Consider, for instance, the sentence-picture matching task. Given that this is a forced-choice task, the most important manipulation is the choice of pictures. Even if the syntactic structure of the stimulus sentence is kept constant, there are many possible error types, and the solution space can clearly influence the outcome. As an example, consider the sentence in (15) and the possible answer sets (each representing a set of pictures) in (16) and (17).

(15) The tall boy kissed the girl.

(16) a. The boy kissed the tall girl.
     b. The tall boy kissed the girl.

(17) a. The tall boy kissed the girl.
     b. The girl kissed the tall boy.

Given (15) as the stimulus sentence and an answer sheet with the pictures whose content is represented in (16), all it takes to answer correctly is to know which of the two depicted characters is tall. In (17), however, one needs to know who did the kissing. We can see, then, how the choice of pictures to define the solution space may influence the outcome: if patients are impaired in a way that enables them to compute adjective-noun relations but does not enable them to compute, say, subject-predicate relations, they might do well when asked to choose between the options in (16) but poorly when asked to choose between those in (17). Similar considerations of course hold for other tasks. An analogous point can be made about types of violation presented to patients in grammaticality judgment tasks. Conceivably, there exist patients whose impairment allows them to detect some violations and makes them insensitive to others. In fact, agrammatic patients exhibit such an effect. (See Linebarger, Schwartz, and Saffran 1983 and the interpretation of their finding in Zurif and Grodzinsky 1983. See also Grodzinsky and Marek 1988.)

Generally, one can imagine a syndrome that allows patients to comprehend some syntactic constructions yet causes them to fail on others. Therefore, if a patient is given one sentential type to interpret, success or failure will not necessarily indicate full intactness, or total disruption, of the language faculty. Thus, the choice of syntactic construction is another major determinant of the aphasic performance level. This we have already seen in discussing the various proposals for describing agrammatism, and we will see it in more detail as the argument proceeds.

Finally, an important issue for the theoretical interpretation of error data is level of performance. The traditional characterization of cognitively impaired people's performance as "good" or "poor" does not suffice for a full interpretation of experimental findings. Since the dependent variable is error rate, the rate itself is extremely important and must be taken into consideration. Take sentence-picture matching experiments, for instance. Usually the task is to assign thematic roles to two noun phrases. Given a sentence like *The girl pushed the boy*, and two pictures (one of a boy pushing a girl, the other of a girl pushing a boy), there may be three possible outcomes: (1) subjects are consistently correct (and determine that the girl did the pushing in our case), in which case their performance level is above chance, (2) they are guessing and give correct answers only half the time (at chance level), or (3) they are consistently wrong (below chance). Both possibilities 2 and 3 count as "poor" performances (or alternatively, the corresponding experimental conditions are "hard," in the terminology of Schwartz et al. 1987). Yet each of them warrants a different interpretation. An account of the findings must be sensitive to this distinction. A comparison of two experimental conditions in which patients performed differently must therefore include two statistics: one that ensures reliable difference between conditions (as is commonly done) and, in addition, one that establishes the relation of each condition to chance level. In this way a precise account of the performances can be constructed.

Three central elements, then, influence the outcome of a comprehension-related experiment: the choice of task, sentential types, and solution space. A schematic analysis of three interpretive tasks, and the difference between them, will make the story clearer. It amounts to a description of the steps minimally involved in each task. In parentheses are the details of each operation necessary for successful performance.

Sentence-picture matching

Sentence
    The tall boy hit the short man.
Pictures
    a tall boy hitting a short man; a short man hitting a tall boy[13]
Task analysis
    hear (read) string → analyze syntactically (*boy* = subject, *man* = object) →
    assign theta-roles (*boy* = agent, *man* = patient) → interpret semantically
    ('boy hit man') → check against solution space for a match → point to ap-
    propriate picture

Sentence
    The tall boy hit the short man.
Pictures
    tall boy hitting short man; short boy hitting tall man
Task analysis
    hear (read) string→ analyze syntactically (*tall* modifies *boy*, *short* modifies
    man)→ interpret semantically ('tall boy hit short man')→ check against sol-
    ution space for a match → point to appropriate picture

Sentence arrangement (anagrams)

Picture
    a boy hitting a man
Sentence fragments
    a boy, hit, a man
Task analysis
    look at picture→ construct semantic representation → arrange cards in what-
    ever way seems possible (NP_1–V–NP_2)→ construct thematic representation of
    string (NP_1 = agent; NP_2 = patient)→ compare with representation. If there is
    a match, keep arrangement; if not, change and start again.

Although this analysis is sketchy, it suffices to show how each task makes different demands on the subject's grammatical abilities. (Tasks differ in other respects, too, but this is the relevant sense for our purposes.) Yet the differences among these tasks are relevant and important only if the problem that patients are suffering impairs their syntactic abilities partially. If the whole language faculty is wiped out—or fully intact—then patients are expected to perform very poorly—or perfectly—in every interpretive task free of time constraints. As it happens, the comprehension abilities of agrammatic aphasic patients indeed appear to be impaired only in part.

3.3.3.1 Patient Groupings   One issue remains to be discussed. It concerns the proper treatment of the variability among patients who fall into the same typological category. It is well known that aphasic patients differ in the severity of their impairment. Moreover, the typology is mostly based on the bedside impressions of clinicians and is not always theoretically motivated. The question is how patients should be grouped, and how differences among members of each clinical category should be interpreted. A clear answer is quite important. Suppose that a claim is advanced, to the effect that a speech production deficit always parallels its comprehension counterpart in some syndrome (see, for example, Caramazza and Zurif 1976). Then a case is found in which only production is impaired (see, for example, Miceli et al. 1983). Will it count as evidence against an "overarching" deficit, as the latter authors argue? Or, rather, are different degrees of severity possible within the same typological category, such that production is impaired first, then comprehension? It seems to me that we should not address this problem from a diagnostic angle. Whether such parallelism is criterial for the diagnosis of a particular syndrome (agrammatism in this case) is a question for clinicians. For them, rehabilitation plans are devised on the basis of classificatory schemas. But for those interested in models of normal language knowledge and use, things are different. In this case the argument should turn on theoretical claims, not on patient groupings per se. If the discovery of parallelism in a patient or group of patients motivates a claim that the same mechanisms underlie both speech production and comprehension, then dissociation between the two in another patient or group of patients should be taken as counterevidence. On the other hand, there may be questions for which it makes no difference at all whether or not the two activities are impaired in the same way. If one investigates, say, the processing of embedded sentences in agrammatism for the sake of understanding how such sentences are represented in the normal head, then one may abstract away from the parallelism debate. This raises an immediate question: Given that the criteria for patient selection are so vague, how should patients be grouped in experimental studies? An extreme position is advanced by Badecker and Caramazza (1985), who assert that grouping patients in neuropsychological studies is simply impossible. They argue that since there is no theoretically motivated criterion for diagnosis, there is no point in patient selection, and given that patients are indeed different, it makes no sense to conduct studies on an undifferentiated population in which variation within the group is extremely high. Moreover, even if coherent, sound criteria existed, they would be useless. They would be used to select patients, and then it would hardly be surprising that the theories from which these criteria were derived were confirmed by experimentation. For Badecker and Caramazza, patient groupings lead to circular argumentation, and they conclude that only case studies should be done in neuropsychology.

This line of reasoning is far from convincing. First, excluding group studies also blocks generalizations and tests of their empirical consequences. A generalization amounts to pooling the patients whose performances fall under it and treating them as a group. Generalizations are the backbone of scientific theories. Yet to prohibit group studies is to prohibit any generalization over data from more than one patient. Thus, an appeal to case studies as the only "defensible methodology" guarantees a dead end. By testing only one patient, the investigator can at best make a claim whose consequences can never be tested. A test would involve another individual, which would immediately amount to a group study. But if such groupings are prohibited, then that is where the investigator is forced to stop. How can we get out of this "logical puzzle" and still keep using groups?

Observe that no area in psychology (or for that matter, any science) enjoys clear a priori criteria to define theoretically relevant domains. We cannot predict in advance how far a theory will go. Domains are defined by theories. If we have a good theory of vision that also explains hearing, smelling, taste, and palpation, then it is a theory about sensory experience and its processing. If—unluckily—we manage to construct a theory about the visual system only, then our domain is narrow. Since there can never be a priori criteria for domain selection, domains should be selected on the basis of intuition as a first step. If intuition tells us that we should look at the visual system as a domain, then our attempt to construct models of it is justified. The same is true in neuropsychology, where no "rigorous criteria" can be set in advance. Badecker and Caramazza thus look for a solution before they even characterize the problem. Agrammatism is a good example in this regard. Long-held intuitions on the part of researchers pointed to its relevance to general issues in language use. And despite some variation within the group of agrammatic patients, the inquiry has led to relevant, testable generalizations. Experience has shown that maintaining the traditional classificatory schema, or refined versions thereof, has borne results, and that tests of undifferentiated aphasic populations, just like case studies, have led nowhere. The conclusion is that the criteria defining the category "agrammatism" have to allow for some *constrained individual variation*. Patients may vary in that some may suffer impairment in, say, both production and comprehension, or only in production; but pooling them together is constrained in that no patient is included whose comprehension is impaired but whose production skills are fully intact. Given that patient groupings are loosely defined, they should be used just as background information, to help the researcher focus on disorders that are relevant to models of normal language knowledge and use.

As another example, suppose a linguistic claim is advanced, based on the observation that in some syndrome the patients can handle active sentences but not passive ones. This hypothetical claim is, say, that the patients cannot properly understand sentences in which nouns are ordered noncanonically. Does a patient who falls into the same diagnostic category, but nevertheless is capable of comprehending both sentence types normally, count as a counterexample? Again, the conditions specified by a theoretical account characterize the performance of a patient population in the limit. In the present case the consequence is that there may never exist a patient who can handle passive but not active constructions. A lesser impairment, though, is permissible under this account. A theoretical claim, if it is concerned with establishing connections among types of syntactic constructions, should take only patients whose performance appears theoretically relevant as empirical evidence. This does not mean that patients are selected to confirm (or disconfirm) theories in a circular fashion, as Badecker and Caramazza argue. This is so because the account in question is constrained, and specifies patterns of impairment that patients may never show (as in the examples given above). In addition, such accounts make predictions that can be tested experimentally. In this example the account predicts that the patients will fail on every sentence type in which nouns are arranged noncanonically, for example, object-cleft sentences (such as *It is the boy who the girl pushed*). Thus, there is nothing circular in this form of reasoning. The "logical puzzle" is not enigmatic at all. (See Zurif, Gardner, and Brownell 1989 and Grodzinsky (forthcoming).)

3.3.4 The Formal Description of Agrammatic Comprehension
In this section I will consider the proper grammatical characterization of the linguistic representations accessible to agrammatic aphasic patients. To begin with two methodological notes: (1) Although I will focus on this single syndrome, if the line of reasoning and methodology I will advocate are correct,

then they hold for any cognitive deficit. (2) Although I will argue that the proposed descriptive generalization characterizes the agrammatic comprehension limitation, whether or not it captures agrammatism only, and no other language deficit, is an open empirical question. Because the data on the syntactic comprehension abilities of Wernicke's, anomic, and conduction patients are so sparse, we are not in a position to make an accurate statement concerning the relation between the deficits in the various aphasias. Deficits might overlap, be a subset one of another, or be totally distinct. To decide the issue would require testing patients from all these categories on the same variety of syntactic constructions. The little available evidence (Caramazza and Zurif 1976; Ansell and Flowers 1982; Grodzinsky 1984b) indicates that, at least for Wernicke's aphasics, the syntactic deficit overlaps with, but differs from, that of the agrammatic aphasics. That is, their performance on some, but not all, syntactic constructions is similar, a fact leading to different linguistic generalizations for each patient group. At this point, then, no data exist to decide the issue either way. This, however, does not diminish the force of the claims about agrammatism, the syndrome on which we focus here.[14]

Consider, first of all, the syntactic abilities of agrammatic aphasics as they emerge from the review just completed. If one looks at the syntactic properties of the sentences presented to the patients in the experiments, at the specific tasks they were presented with, and at their error types and rates, it turns out that from a syntactic point of view their impairment is partial: they are able to assign correct interpretations to, and correctly judge the acceptability of, certain construction types, while failing on others. A description of their loss, then, would require fine-grained grammatical distinctions. It is only such phenomena that make neuropsychology interesting for linguists, and vice versa.

3.3.4.1 Some Data and What They Suggest This survey of empirical results focuses on the syntactic properties of the sentences presented to agrammatic patients, while keeping other factors fixed. All the sentences are reversible semantically, the types of response and solution spaces are such that the patient's task is always to assign theta-roles to two NPs in a clause, and the dependent variable measured is performance level (percentage error) and its relation to chance. Two kinds of performance results are to be found in the literature: on some syntactic constructions patients perform at an above-chance level of accuracy, whereas on others they perform at chance level.[15] In passive sentences, such as (18a), the aphasic is supposed to associate the agent (or actor) role with the last noun phrase (NP) in the sequence and the theme (acted-upon) role with the first NP, whereas in its active counterpart (18b) the situation is reversed.

(18) a. The girl was pushed by the boy.
    b. The girl pushed the boy.

It turns out that on passives agrammatics perform at chance; that is, they are uncertain about the interpretation of these constructions and therefore guess. On actives, however, they perform above chance, virtually normally (see among others, Schwartz, Saffran, and Marin 1980; Caplan and Futter 1986; Grodzinsky et al. 1988). Similar results have been been found regarding object versus subject relatives (Caramazza and Zurif 1976; Grodzinsky 1984b, 1989; Wulfeck 1984), exemplified in (19), and for object versus subject clefts (Caplan and Futter 1986), exemplified in (20). In both cases agrammatic patients perform at chance level on the object (a) construction and at an above-chance level on its subject (b) counterpart.

(19) a. The girl who the boy is pushing is tall. (object)[16]
    b. The girl who is pushing the boy is tall. (subject)

(20) a. It is the girl who the boy is pushing. (object)
    b. It is the girl who is pushing the boy. (subject)

It must be stressed that the error analysis performed in these experiments differs substantially from the usual grammatical analysis. Whereas grammatical analysis is based on statements about sentences such as "S is grammatical," "S is ill formed," and "S is ambiguous," the analysis of interpretive errors examines statements such as "The patient's comprehension of S was above chance" and "The patient's comprehension of S was at chance" (alternatively, "The patient's judgment of the grammaticality of S was accurate 70 percent of the time," and so on). In testing comprehension, we are mainly looking at three performance types: above-, below-, and at-chance levels. Thus, it is extremely important to notice that all the instances we have looked at so far exhibit only two performance types—random (chance-level) and correct (above-chance)—even though there is a third logically possible type: below-chance, namely, consistent *inversion* of thematic roles. Any account of these findings must not only predict the observed outcomes. It must also rule out the other possible, yet unobserved, result. None of the traditional descriptions do so. Nor do they account for the sharp (rather than gradual) rise in performance between the (a) and (b) cases in (19) and (20).

    The next stage is to state a generalization that will distinguish the constructions that yielded above-chance performance from the rest, a statement going beyond the data. Then such a hypothesis can be subjected to further empirical tests. Prima facie, it seems that syntactic variables will have to be invoked. Indeed, the presentation of the data so far has not been accidental and is intended to lead to a syntactic generalization. The central idea is that a single syntactic factor distinguishes sentence types that patients interpret correctly from those that they interpret at chance level. This distinction turns on syntactic movement.

3.3.4.2 The Syntax of the Relevant Constructions
The essentials of the Government-Binding (GB) Theory of syntax were presented in chapter 2. To recap briefly: The grammar comprises (1) several levels of representation, (2) rules, and (3) constraints. Every sentence in every language is associated with representations at each level, which are subject to a variety of well-formedness conditions and are related to one another by rules. A sentence is well formed if and only if all of its representations are well formed. D-structure and S-structure, which are two of these levels, are related to one another by a transformational rule known as Move-Alpha, which can move constituents around.

Now let us look at the aspects of the constructions under discussion that are crucial for the analysis of agrammatism.

Consider passive first. Assuming that the transformational rule of Move-Alpha is never obligatory and that the D-structure representation of a passive sentence is as in (21a), some principles must be invoked to force *John,* the NP in object position, to move to subject position. Recall that the Case Filter excludes representations containing lexical NPs that are not assigned Case. If passivization of a verb is taken to be an operation that entails insertion of passive morphology, absorption of Case, and dethematization of the subject (that is, a process in which the subject position loses its theta-role), then the consequences for the passive construction are as follows. The lexical NP in object position in (21a) will not have Case. It will have to move to the (Cased) subject position, leaving a trace behind. In its new position this NP will not have an independent theta-role, since this position is now nonthematic (having been dethematized by passivization). The NP will now inherit the theta-role assigned to its trace, by virtue of the index they share (or by virtue of their being members of the same chain). This sequence of operations is demonstrated by the abbreviated representations in (21), where *e* stands for a base-generated empty position and *t* is an empty position resulting from movement:

(21) a. [e] was pushed John   (D-structure representation)
     b. [John]$_i$ was pushed t_i (S-structure representation)

Several principles of grammar interact to govern the distribution of NP-traces. Some of these were discussed in chapter 2. For further discussion, see Van Riemsdijk and Williams 1986 and Bouchard 1984.

Relative clauses have some similar properties, though overall their syntactic structure is somewhat different. They, too, are derived transformationally. In this case, however, the trace is a *wh*-trace (making this construction pattern with questions, among others), and the moved element moves from its original site to Comp position. The element in Comp, which may or may not be overt, functions like an operator that binds a variable. Indeed, *wh*-traces are believed to be variables. The relation between the relative clause and its head (the NP to which it refers) is a predication relation, whereby the relative clause is predicated of its head. In the example in (22), which is the S-structure representation of a center-embedded object relative (*cats who mice eat are happy*), movement takes place from object position in the relative clause (marked by NP_3) to Comp, and this clause is predicated of the head, NP_1. Here too, an NP in Comp position (functioning as an operator that binds the trace—a variable) inherits a thematic role from the trace in object position. This fact will be important for the characterization of agrammatism I propose below.

(22)

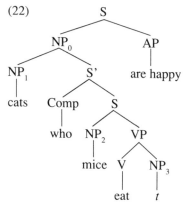

Though quite different, relative clauses like the one in (22) and passives like the one in (21) are similar in that (1) they involve traces in their syntactic represen-tations at S-structure and (2) these traces play a mediating role in the process of theta-role assignment.

Traces are crucial for semantic interpretation. Theta-roles like agent, theme, source, and goal (see, for example, Gruber 1965; Jackendoff 1972), which play a central part in the construction of the semantic representation of a sentence, are always assigned to syntactic positions, regardless of the identity of the assignee. As we saw in chapter 2, a lexical category assigning theta-roles has a represen-tation in its lexical entry called a theta-grid (Stowell 1981; Higginbotham 1985), which specifies the number and identity of the assignees with which it is to be associated. Theta-roles are assigned under a restricted set of structural relations, and when the requirements are met, the assignment is "read off" the lexical entry of the assigner, and the assignees "discharge" the assigner (Higginbotham 1985).

Crucially, this process is defined over syntactic positions and is insensitive to the content with which they are filled. It is indifferent to whether a position is filled with lexical material or empty, as long as it is structurally represented. If a thematic position is filled with a lexical NP (for example, the subject or object of an active sentence), then this NP receives its theta-role directly (the subject is usually assigned a role by the VP, and the object by the verb). If a thematic position contains a trace, this trace is assigned a theta-role, which it transmits to its antecedent (the NP moved from this position by Move-Alpha). In the two constructions under discussion the verb assigns the theta-role of theme to the position occupied by the trace in the passive, object-relative, and object-cleft cases. This theta-role is transmitted from the trace to its antecedent NP, since they are linked by virtue of the index they share (in GB terminology, they form a "chain").

The following examples illustrate additional construction types for which there are data from agrammatism. The forms given are their S-structure representations, where all the currently irrelevant information is suppressed.

(23) a. $[_{NP}$ the girl$]_i$ was pushed $[_{NP} t]_i$ by $[_{NP}$ the boy$]$
     b. $[_{NP}$ the girl$]$ pushed $[_{NP}$ the boy$]$

(24) a. $[_{NP}$ the girl$]_i$ who $[_{NP}$ the boy$]$ is pushing $[_{NP} t]_i$ is tall
     b. $[_{NP}$ the girl$]_i$ who $[_{NP} t]_i$ is pushing $[_{NP}$ the boy$]$ is tall
     c. show me $[_{NP}$ the girl$]_i$ who $[_{NP}$ the boy$]$ is pushing $[_{NP} t]_i$
     d. show me $[_{NP}$ the girl$]_i$ who $[_{NP} t]_i$ is pushing $[_{NP}$ the boy$]$

(25) a. it is $[_{NP}$ the girl$]_i$ who $[_{NP}$ the boy$]$ is pushing $[_{NP} t]_i$
     b. it is $[_{NP}$ the girl$]_i$ who $[_{NP} t]_i$ is pushing $[_{NP}$ the boy$]$

A trace appears in the object position of all the (a) and (c) cases, but not in the (b) and (d) cases. In the latter, if there is a trace in the S-structure representation (as in (24b,d) and (25b)), it is in the subject position. This contrast in structural properties correlates with chance (on the (a) and (c) cases) versus correct (on the (b) and (d) cases) performance. Observationally, then, chance performance is attested just in case the S-structure representation of a stimulus sentence contains a trace in object position.

3.3.4.3 A Descriptive Generalization
The proposed account of agrammatic comprehension patterns is based on the observation that from a syntactic point of view, all the sentences on which the patients performed at chance level share one property: the derivation of their S-structure representations from D-structure is transformational. Specifically, they all involve movement from

object position, and consequently their S-structure representations contain a trace in this position.

By contrast, the constructions on which the agrammatic subjects performed correctly do not have this property. If there is a trace in their S-structure representation, it is in the subject position.

The next step is to state a generalization. Yet a problem immediately arises: if we say that every sentence that contains a trace would lead to chance performance in agrammatic comprehension, we cover subject relatives and subject clefts, which are transformational (at least on some analyses; see below). We need to pick out only the sentences that have a trace in object position. A difference in the thematic properties of subjects and objects (at least those associated with agentive verbs, the only ones at issue right now) may help: in active sentences subjects are agents, whereas objects are themes or patients. The interaction of the two properties just mentioned leads to a generalization.

Capitalizing on the preceding observations, it remains to state the generalization itself. Syntactic representations in agrammatism are generally intact, except in the two respects noted in (26).

(26) a. *Trace Deletion*
   All traces are deleted from S-structure level.

   b. *Default Principle*
   NPs that do not receive a theta-role syntactically are assigned a default theta-role. Or, stated more precisely in terms of GB Theory: NPs in nonthematic positions are under the scope of some Default Principle that associates a theta-role to every nonthematic position.

For the moment the Default Principle will be assumed to operate in the manner first proposed by Bever (1970) and then adopted by many others studying adult psycholinguistics and language acquisition (for example, Slobin and Bever 1982; Hakuta 1981). That is, once it is invoked, then (regardless of what sentence grammar would dictate) it will by default associate the clause-initial position with the role of agent in SVO languages like English, and the postverbal position with the role of patient. For now, the Default Principle is taken to be nonlinguistic. The association of roles to positions does not come from grammatical principles; rather, it is invoked when the grammar fails, and it is based on the speaker's general, nonlinguistic knowledge (for example, that in English the subject position is filled by an agent most of the time). Later, when we carefully reexamine this assumption, we will see that it plays a crucial role in the argument.

Granting these two assumptions, Trace Deletion and the Default Principle, all the data are predicted: in the (a) and (c) cases in (23)–(25) the first NP (*the girl*) does not receive a theta-role configurationally. This is so because the trace it is associated with is deleted (by Trace Deletion), and it is this trace that would have served as a link for the transmission of a theta-role to the NP in question. This NP is thus "dangling," from a thematic point of view. But notice that it is in a nonthematic position. This puts it under the scope of the Default Principle, which assigns it the role of agent, because it is clause-initial. The other NP in these clauses (*the boy*) is assigned the role of agent directly by the VP, because it is in the subject position of its clause. The assignment of the same theta-role to two NPs creates a conflict that results in chance-level performance. The Default Principle, then, operates here like a cleanup hitter hitting into a double play: it is invoked in order to salvage a deficient representation, but because of the circumstances its application results in a representation that leads the patient to guessing.

Now consider the (b) and (d) cases. Their geometry is different, and therefore the conflict between the Default Principle and the normal assignment of theta-roles does not arise. The active case (23b) contains no traces; hence, no interpretive problem should arise. In the (b) and (d) cases of (24) and (25) the first NP is assigned the agent role by default, yet this is precisely the role it would have received had it been linked to its trace. It follows, then, that although the agrammatic patients answer correctly in these cases, they do so for the wrong reasons; namely, their correct performance is achieved by default, in spite of the deficient, traceless representation. Their successful interpretation of these sentences is due to an accidental overlap between the role assigned by the Default Principle and the role that should have been transmitted through the trace.

The assignment of theta-roles in agrammatism to the sentences discussed, and the performances this arrangement predicts, are given in (27)–(29). The motivation for this assignment is given in parentheses: S signifies structural assignment of the theta-role, D signifies assignment via the Default Principle. Deletion of traces is signified by *.

(27) a. [the girl] was pushed * by [the boy]   (chance)
          agent (D)   agent (S)

    b. [the girl] pushed [the boy]   (above chance)
        agent (S)   theme (S)

(28) a. [the girl] who [the boy] is pushing * is tall   (chance)
          agent (D)   agent (S)

    b. [the girl] who * is pushing [the boy] is tall   (above chance)
        agent (D)   theme (S)

c. show me [the girl] who [the boy] is pushing *   (chance)
         | |
      agent (D)   agent (S)

d. show me [the girl] who * is pushing [the boy]   (above chance)
         | |
      agent (D)   theme (S)[17]

(29) a. it is [the girl] who [the boy] is pushing *   (chance)
         | |
      agent (D)   agent (S)

b. it is [the girl] who * is pushing [the boy]   (above chance)
         | |
      agent (D)   theme (S)

The predictions can be verified by comparing the position of the trace at S-structure in (23)–(25) to the predictions and assignment of theta-roles in the corresponding sentences of (27)–(29). Above-chance performance appears either where no transformational operation takes place (see (27b)) or where Move-Alpha extracts an NP from subject position, leaving behind a trace (see (28b,d), (29b)). In these two instances the resulting thematic representation contains one agent and one theme, and these roles represent the correct thematic arrangement. Chance performance always appears where there are two agents (see (27a), (28a,c), (29a)). This thematic structure appears where the S-structure representation of a sentence contains a trace in object position.

In sum, what is crucial for predicting aberrant and normal performance is the relationship between the normally assigned theta-role and the default assignment. The default strategy may assign the NP under its scope a theta-role that is either identical to or different from the theta-role that is grammatically assigned to this position. Should the two roles be the same, then normal, above-chance performance is predicted, as with subject gaps. On the other hand, should the two roles be different, then aberrant performance is predicted, as with object gaps and passives.

So far, this description appears to be correct. It is compatible with all the data at hand. Next let us examine some of its properties.

3.3.4.4 Some Noteworthy Properties of the Proposal   First, it is almost meaningless to say that the Trace Deletion–Default Principle account is a *theory* of agrammatism, in light of the introductory remarks about deficit descriptions and their role in cognitive science. It is a descriptive generalization that captures given data in an economical way, while capitalizing on distinctions provided by a well-motivated theory of syntactic representation. It does so by making a minimal number of assumptions about the agrammatic deficit. Only in this way can it later be tied to theoretical issues.

Second, this account differs sharply from connectionist and British information-processing accounts discussed in chapter 1. It focuses on representations,
not processes, whereas the other two approaches focus only on processes,
without tying them to knowledge (grammatical or other) at all. These accounts
are mainly concerned with the differences among channels of communication
that humans possess, whereas here the chief concern is grammatical ability. To
this end, a well-articulated theory of grammatical representation is used as a
discovery procedure of the pattern of selectivity in the aphasic deficit. Stating a
generalization over observed patterns allows one to derive clear predictions for
heretofore unobserved aspects of the deficit and put them to empirical test. If this
description is correct, then both connectionism and most information-processing
models are immediately falsified, because they are incapable of accounting for
the comprehension patterns that distinguish among syntactic types (as indeed
recorded in the studies of agrammatics that have been reviewed).

Third, the present account capitalizes on the interaction between general,
nonlinguistic knowledge and knowledge of language, both of which are part and
parcel of the act of communication. Yet it is stated in a way that does not blur the
distinction between the two knowledge sources.

3.3.4.5 Extending the Data Base   We have seen how the assumptions we
have made result in agrammatic representations of several construction types,
where traces are deleted. The interaction of the Default Principle with the
remainder of the syntactic representation available to the agrammatic patient
results in a thematic representation that may or may not be correct, depending on
the syntactic construction in question.

This proposal, however, was based on sentences containing agentive verbs
only—that is, verbs whose theta-grid contains the role of agent. But there are
other verb types (compare *receive, fear, seem,* and so on). And, although it was
made clear that a syntactic classification of constructions is necessary, the
strategy assumed to be invoked by default was quite generic in nature. This
focuses our attention on the interaction between the Default Principle and the
thematic properties of the verb in question. Is the principle sensitive to thematic
properties, or will it assign the agent role even in contexts where this role would
not normally have been assigned? With this question in mind it is naturally
interesting to look at the nonagentive verbs. They can serve as a test that will
distinguish the default strategy proposed above from another, linguistically
based one, sensitive to thematic properties of verbs. So far the default assignment
has referred to a "canonical" arrangement that is discovered through observing
statistical preponderances in language use. For example, the usual, most frequent

order of theta-roles in English is agent-action-theme. According to the proposed strategy, arguments are assigned the agent and theme roles even if their predicate is a verb that does not have these roles in its theta-grid. Were this strategy to apply in active sentences with verbs like *hit*, as in (30a), all would be well, because the format of the verbs conforms with this principle. Were it to apply with verbs such as *hate,* as in (30b), however, it would still assign the theta-role of agent to the subject, and so on, contrary to the actual thematic properties of these verbs.

(30) *Thematic representations with a cognitively based default strategy*

            Grammatical assignment

    agent   theme   experiencer theme
     | | | |
a. John hit Bill   b. John hated Mary
     | | | |
    agent   theme   agent   theme

            Default Assignment

More significantly, thematic representations for passive in agrammatism would now be as shown in (31).

(31) a. Bill was hit by John   b. Mary was hated by John
      | | | |
    agent   agent   agent   experiencer

The theta-roles in (31) are assigned as before. In (31a) agent is assigned to *Bill* by the Default Principle and to *John* by the grammar. In (31b) agent is assigned to *Mary* by default, and experiencer is assigned to *John* by the grammar. (Normal assignment of theta-roles takes place in the by-phrase, by assumption.) Thus, the account predicts that the subjects of all passives in agrammatism are assigned the role agent, regardless of the thematic properties of their verbs.

Yet there is another possible formulation of the Default Principle. The knowledge on which it is based may not stem from observations about frequencies of occurrence. Rather, it may be linguistic: the theta-grid of the verb itself. According to this proposal, in the default situation the preverbal NP of a verb like *hit* would be assigned the theta-role agent, the preverbal NP of *hate* would be assigned experiencer, while the postverbal NPs would have the same thematic labels as before.

(32) *Thematic representations with a linguistically based default strategy*
    a. John was hit by Bill   b. Mary was hated by John
        | | | |
    agent   agent   experiencer   experiencer

Now compare the thematic representations in (32) to those in (31). The agent-first strategy always assigns the clause-initial position the agent role, whereas the strategy based on the theta-grid assigns it the role it finds in the lexicon; thus, for a verb like *hate* the clause-initial NP *Mary* receives the role agent in (31b) and experiencer in (32b). This difference between (31b) and (32b) surely leads to different predictions. Since the data reported so far cannot decide this issue (the representations in (31a) and (32a) are identical), the next step is to look at "experiencer" and other nonagentive verbs, to hone the formulation of the Default Principle and discover whether it is based on cognitive or linguistic knowledge.

To test these verbs, three colleagues and I conducted an experiment in which we assessed the sensitivity of aphasic patients to sentences containing arguments with a variety of thematic identities (Grodzinsky et al. 1988). Unlike previous analyses of the use of the linear strategy in aphasia, in which only basic agentive verbs had been employed, we attempted to provide a systematic contrast between sentences containing agentive and nonagentive predicates. Two sets of contrasts were examined. In one condition the contrast was established by manipulating the animacy of the arguments as in (33) and (34).

(33) The priest covers the nun.

(34) The book covers the newspaper.

The verb is ambiguous in (33), having potentially an agentive reading and a nonagentive reading. In (34), however, only a nonagentive reading is available. Thus, only in (33) could the subject be assigned the theta-role agent. The second experimental condition involved the class of so-called psychological verbs, which includes *admire* and *understand*.[18] These verbs were chosen because even though they must be coupled with animate arguments, they do not normally assign agent to these arguments but instead assign a distinct theta-role, usually denoted experiencer. The distinction between agent and experiencer can be seen in the contrast between (35a) and (35b).

(35) a. *He admired her on purpose.
     b. He murdered her on purpose.

Actually, psychological verbs allow agentive readings under some highly restricted conditions. Still, for expository purposes the contrast between agentive and nonagentive sentences may be considered to be of two types. The first involves sentences containing ambiguous verbs where the agentive or nonagentive reading is determined by the animacy or inanimacy of the subject. The second involves sentences that differ in agentivity because of thematic properties of the verb itself, animacy being kept constant. In all cases in this experiment this contrast was coupled with a syntactic manipulation: an active-passive contrast.

This experiment also assessed the patients' overall grammatical knowledge, knowledge that might be obscured if the more usual sentence-picture matching task had been used. It did so by using a sentence-arrangement (anagram) task, which, unlike the sentence-picture matching task, allowed us to see whether, and to what extent, these patients would order two nouns together, a performance that would indicate a severe syntactic loss. Thus, shown a picture of some relation between two people or objects (a relation always compatible with the verb types described above), patients were asked to arrange sentence fragments into a sentence that correctly described the picture. Two comparisons were made: performance on the sentences containing agentive verbs was compared to performance on those containing nonagentive verbs, and performance on active constructions was compared to performance on passive constructions. This experiment thus had the eight conditions listed in table 3.1.

Table 3.1

	Condition	Example
1	Basic agentive active	The policeman stops the soldier.
2	Basic agentive passive	The soldier is stopped by the policeman.
3	Ambiguous agentive active (animate)	The priest covers the nun.
4	Ambiguous agentive passive (animate)	The nun is covered by the priest.
5	Nonagentive active (inanimate)	The book covers the newspaper.
6	Nonagentive passive (inanimate)	The newspaper is covered by the book.
7	Psychological active	The man admires the woman.
8	psychological passive	The woman is admired by the man.

In each trial the patients were given one picture and three sentence fragments. Their task was to arrange the fragments so that they matched the picture. Thus, for a sentence such as *The policeman is stopped by the soldier*, the fragments were *the policeman*, *is stopped by*, and *the soldier*. Since we were interested in the theta-role assignment, our fragmentation did not take considerations of constituency into account. The pictures were clear line drawings. Those containing situations corresponding to the psychological verbs were carefully drawn and thoroughly tested with matched-normal controls beforehand to ensure that the mental state displayed was easily identifiable.

The results were very clear. First, the patients virtually never arranged the cards so as to create an ungrammatical sequence. In some cases, as we will see, their interpretation was incorrect, but overall they showed a deficit that was indeed restricted to theta-role assignment in certain sentential types. This result clearly indicates that the patients were aware of the concept "sentence." Their solution space included options like *the man the woman is admired by*, that being a possible ordering of the cards. Yet they never made such errors. This falsifies accounts of agrammatic comprehension according to which these patients are unaware of phrasal syntax.

Second, on all the active sentences (odd-numbered conditions in table 3.1) they performed well above chance, demonstrating an ability to appreciate the syntactic parameters relevant to theta-role assignment. Third, patients performed at chance level on the agentive and nonagentive passives (conditions 2, 4, 6). This result not only replicates those of previous experiments but also shows that agentivity is not a factor determining aberrant performance in these constructions. Finally, the psychological passives (condition 8) yielded below-chance performance; that is, the patients consistently inverted the theta-roles in these sentences.

The experiment thus yielded a three-way grouping of conditions, clustered according to performance types, each group differing significantly from the others. These results show, to a first approximation, that the idea of looking at verbs according to their thematic properties led to interesting results—a very fine breakdown pattern. But they also indicate that we should go back to the drawing board and revise the account. A simplistic view of the Default Principle is not enough.

3.3.4.6   Extending the Account   Consider first those verbs termed "ambiguous nonagentive" and the normal theta-role assignment in constructions containing them.

(36) [The book] is covered by [the newspaper].
         | |
       theme   instrument

If Trace Deletion and application of the "nonlinguistic" Default Principle operate here too, then for the agrammatic subjects, theta-roles would have to be assigned as shown in (37).

(37) [The book] is covered by [the newspaper].
         | |
       agent   instrument

This operation would be a result of the "blind" application of the Default Principle: it would assign agenthood to *any* clause-initial NP that does not have a theta-role. This account, however, runs into empirical as well as conceptual difficulties. To examine these, we will have to refer to the theta-grid and the labels of its arguments, as discussed in chapter 2. Recall the Thematic Hierarchy Condition, which specifies the order of saliency among thematic identities shown in (38).

(38) 1. Agent
2. Goal, source, instrument, experiencer
3. Theme

Issues of hierarchy among theta-roles arise here for the first time. In the cases examined so far, aberrant performance resulted from the presence of two identical theta-roles in the same sentence. But now we have a new situation, where two different theta-roles (not identical to the normally assigned ones) appear. When we take the Thematic Hierarchy Condition into account, new predictions emerge. Suppose that the Default Principle applied to (36), yielding the thematic representation in (37). Patients would then make consistent reversal errors in nonagentive passive sentences like (36), interpreting them as if they were active. This would happen because the subject of these sentences (agent) would now be higher on the hierarchy than the object (theme). Consistent reversal would show up as below-chance level of performance. This, of course, is not found: the patients in our experiment performed at chance level on nonagentive passives. Notice, however, that this account forces the assignment of an agent role to an inanimate noun. Yet agents can only be animate, and surely this knowledge is spared in agrammatism, as exemplified by the patients' ability to distinguish between "semantically irreversible" sentences with inanimate agents and "implausible" sentences with animate ones (Caramazza and Zurif 1976; see Grodzinsky and Marek 1988 for a reinterpretation of this finding).

Clearly, in order to be descriptively adequate we must modify our assumptions so that, in addition to accounting for the previously collected data, they will result in a thematic representation that predicts chance performance with the "ambiguous" verbs in the experimental task. Such a representation must assign identical theta-roles to both the subject and the object of nonagentive passive verbs (or at least theta-roles that are on a par on the Thematic Hierarchy) yet allow for normal theta-role assignments in the active case. This could be done by assuming a Default Principle like (39) that is sensitive to the thematic properties of the verb. This was one of the two options considered above.

(39) *Default Principle*
Assign an NP that did not receive a theta-role syntactically (more precisely: assign every nonthematic position) the theta-role that occupies the corresponding position in the theta-grid of the verb.

Here is how this algorithm works. Theta-grids are linearly organized constructs. As shown in (40), the algorithm in (39) identifies an NP without a theta-role, examines its linear position in the clause, checks the corresponding position in the theta-grid (the external argument), and assigns the NP the label it found in that position.

(40) a. John was killed by Bill.
      | |
     *   agent

    b. hit: <agent _____ theme> (theta-grid)

    c. *John* has no thematic label.
      John is the clause-initial NP.
      Agent is the theta-role assigned to the theta-grid initial (external) argument.
      Therefore
      Agent is assigned to *John*.

    d. John was killed by Bill.
       | |
    agent   agent

(40a) is the thematic representation of the sentence as the (deficient) grammar analyzes it. According to the Trace-Deletion Hypothesis, NPs in nonthematic positions (that is, those moved by a transformation) would not have a theta-role in agrammatism, and they would trigger the Default Principle. (40b) and (40c) describe the operation of the Default Principle, and (40d) is the resulting agrammatic thematic representation.

This formulation gives the desired results for active and passive constructions in agrammatism. In active sentences all the roles are assigned syntactically (recall that the representation is intact except for traces, which do not appear in the representation of active sentences). In agentive passive sentences the subject should receive a theta-role by default. Since the subject is associated with the agent role in the theta-grid, the subject of the passive will be assigned the agent role. However, the object will also be assigned agent. Thus, chance performance is predicted. The same holds for nonagentive passive sentences, because the Default Principle is sensitive to the thematic properties of the predicate. The preverbal position in the theta-grid of nonagentive verbs contains exactly the label that the *by*-object receives syntactically. And it is the same label that the Default Principle assigns to the subject. This account therefore predicts chance performance, which is indeed found. (41) gives the resulting representation.

(41) [The book] is covered by [the newspaper].
      | |
   instrument   instrument

This move is actually desirable conceptually. We are in effect claiming that properties of the verb in question determine the identity of the role the default strategy assigns to the nonthematic position. Recall the bizarre prediction that the agent-first default strategy makes for verbs with nonagentive readings. In a task that requires matching sentences to (or constructing an anagram from) pictures, it makes no sense to assign the agent role to an argument that can never be agentive for semantic reasons, that is, an inanimate entity. It is therefore reasonable to assume that even though heuristic strategies are stated over positions, they are nonetheless sensitive to the thematic properties of the assigner involved. The reformulation is descriptively adequate.

Having accounted for nonagentives, we can move on to the psychological verbs. We will see that the reformulation of the Default Principle is insufficient to account for these and that further modification is needed. Recall that agrammatic performance on passive sentences with psychological verbs in the Grodzinsky et al. experiment was significantly below chance. That is, the aphasic subjects consistently interpreted these sentences incorrectly. Had they performed at chance, we could have attributed their responses to the application of the strategy as stated above: since these predicates canonically assign the role of experiencer to their subjects, the subject of the passive (*the man* in (42)) would be assigned an experiencer role. The oblique object (*the woman* in (42)) would also be assigned this role, by the normal process of theta-role assignment.

(42) [The man] is adored by [the woman].
   experiencer   experiencer

Here, however, we run into a descriptive difficulty. The consequence of (42) is chance performance. Yet the aphasic patients performed below chance level, consistently inverting the roles in psychological passives. Thus, the Default Principle now appears descriptively inadequate, and we must consider how it can be appropriately modified. Unlike the earlier finding of chance performance, this result cannot be explained by appealing to identity of theta-roles vis à vis the Thematic Hierarchy. It can be derived only if the role assigned to the subject NP is higher in the hierarchy than the role assigned to the object.

Consider the possible relations among theta-roles in a sentence and their consequences for performance levels observed in agrammatism. Chance performance is predicted when the theta-roles assigned to the NPs in question are identical (or at least equal on the Thematic Hierarchy), and below-chance performance is predicted whenever the normal and pathological assignments are inverse (or at least have the opposite hierarchical order). For the construction shown in (43), where X and Y are theta-roles, all these arrangements are illustrated in table 3.2.

(43) NP...NP
  X Y

Table 3.2

Normal assignment	Pathological assignment	Performance level
X < Y	X < Y	above chance
X < Y	X = Y	at chance
X < Y	X > Y	below chance

X and Y are theta-roles
>, <, and = are relative orders on the Thematic Hierarchy

In its current formulation the Default Principle accounts for above-chance and at-chance results. We must now modify it in order to account for the below-chance responses found with psychological verbs. From these considerations it follows that if we want to keep the general form of the description and account as well for the results with psychological passives, we must modify the description in such a way that the patient's thematic representation for sentences containing psychological verbs has an agent, because agent is the only role higher than experiencer on the Thematic Hierarchy. This modification is shown in (44).

(44) [The man] is adored by [the woman].

X = theme Y = experiencer ($X < Y$)   normal
X = agent Y = experiencer ($X > Y$)   aphasic

This is the only way for the Trace-Deletion Hypothesis to predict below-chance performance. More generally, above-chance performance is predicted for thematic representations in which the hierarchical order of the normally assigned theta-roles matches that of the pathologically assigned ones.[19] But this would mean that, with respect to the Default Principle, we are back to square one. We have considered two versions of this principle: one that assigns roles based on the speaker's experience, by observing statistical regularities in the appearance of noun phrases with respect to linear positions in strings; and another that picks a theta-role by consulting the lexical representation of the verb in question. The data from psychological verbs suggests that the former version is correct: if the role of agent is assigned to the subject of a passive verb regardless of the thematic properties of the particular verb in the stimulus sentence, then the experimental results are accounted for. Yet now we have a serious problem. The patients' performance on the psychological passives suggests a formulation of the Default Principle that blocks its access to linguistic knowledge and allows it to rely only on general cognitive knowledge acquired through experience. Yet their performance on other nonagentive passives suggests the opposite. Is there a reasonable way out of this bind?

We are confronted with two issues here: the descriptive issue we have been discussing, and a conceptual one. The conceptual issue turns on the difference between the two conceivable types of default strategies. If the strategy relies on linguistic knowledge, then it follows that grammatical resources are available not only to grammatical processes but also to compensatory heuristics. If the strategy is divorced from linguistic knowledge, however, then it follows that there is a clear partition between language and general cognition. This point will be central in chapter 5, where we will examine the relevance of neuropsychological findings to the thesis of the modularity of language.

Returning to the descriptive issue, we must now reformulate the Default Principle. In fact, we are forced to return to the version that identifies theta-roles by their linear position, not by their relation to positions on the theta-grid—in other words, the version that captures the data from agentive and psychological verbs. But what about the nonagentive passives? If descriptive adequacy is to be achieved there, the role assigned to the subject must come from the same level in the hierarchy as the role assigned to the *by*-object, and this will not be the case if the Default Principle identifies the subject as agent. Yet notice that all subjects in the nonagentive cases are inanimate. This is how the nonagentive reading was forced in those sentences. It is thus not particularly surprising that the assignment of the agent theta-role was not effective. Inanimates can never be agents, as attested by the contrast in (45).

(45) a. The mother covered the child on purpose/intentionally.

   b. *The newspaper covered the book on purpose/intentionally.

We can now capitalize on this fact, by requiring a match in semantic properties between the role the strategy assigns and the assignee (the subject of the passive). If there is a match (for instance, if the theta-role is agent and the NP is animate), then the role is assigned; if not, then the Default Principle picks a theta-role from the next lower level in the Thematic Hierarchy (in this case, instrument). This final formulation of the principle is shown in (46).

(46) *Default Principle* (final version)

   If a lexical NP has no theta-role (that is, it is in a nonthematic position), assign it the theta-role that is canonically associated with the position it occupies, *unless* this assignment is blocked. In this case assign it a role from the next lower level in the Thematic Hierarchy.

This formulation accounts for all the data. In agentive passives both the object and the subject are assigned the agent role, the former grammatically and the latter by the Default Principle, resulting in chance performance. In psychological passives the subject is assigned the agent role and the object the experiencer role, resulting in below-chance performance.[20] Finally, in nonagentive passives the object and subject are both assigned the instrument role, resulting in chance performance.[21]

In its final version the Default Principle is reminiscent of the learning strategy Pinker (1984) has proposed for children: syntactic positions are linked to theta-roles, regardless of the thematic composition of the verb in question. The strategy proposed here has two steps. First it attempts to assign a role to the NP in question automatically, ignoring the assigner. If this assignment is aborted because of a mismatch in semantic properties (that is, if the assignee is inanimate), then the Default Principle picks a role from the next lower level in the Thematic Hierarchy, to match whatever semantic properties the NP has. The Default Principle is invoked only after grammatical analysis has been found to be insufficient; only then may it look at the semantic properties of the thematically "dangling" NP, to which it assigns a theta-role. Thus, we abandon the account that tied the default theta-role assignment to the theta-grid of the verb, because of its descriptive inadequacy.

Note, incidentally, that the agent role assigned by the grammar differs from the agent role assigned by the Default Principle, in that the former is a grammatically based theta-role and the latter is a semantic role based on world knowledge. Yet clearly there must be a close correspondence between the two, if sentence grammar is ever to help language users in interpretation and action. It is for this reason that I have been referring to them as if they were identical.

Having formulated the strategy, we must now question its motivation. Are there any reasons for invoking it, or is it merely stipulation?

The fact that default assignment may go against grammatical principles is compatible with the conclusion that it does not follow from knowledge of grammar. (For further discussion, see chapter 5, and for opposing views, see Grodzinsky and Johnson 1985 and Frazier, Clifton, and Randall 1983.) Bever (1970), for one, though formulating strategies quite differently, attempted to find motivation for each of them in other cognitive domains. I will not do this here. At this point I can say only that it seems plausible to assume that people attempt to fix the reference of linguistic expressions even when grammatical information is insufficient. Witness, for example, our ability to decipher many ungrammatical sequences, or sentences masked by noise, just by context or by relying on statistical regularities in language use. It is not surprising that aphasics should invoke these abilities. What is interesting, though, is that the proposed account points to cases where the use of strategies goes against the patients' interest and actually confuses them.

In sum, the extension of the original account of agrammatic comprehension, stated in (47), is intended to cover cases involving nonagentive theta-roles. It assumes the same deficient grammatical representation as the original account but refines the nongrammatical principle that is invoked to augment the incomplete syntactic representation for interpretive purposes.

(47) The S-structure representation underlying agrammatic comprehension lacks traces. In interpretation, a Default Principle is invoked that is defined as follows:

If a lexical NP has no theta-role (that is, it is in a nonthematic position), assign it the theta-role that is canonically associated with the position it occupies, *unless* this assignment is blocked. In this case assign it a role from the next lower level in the Thematic Hierarchy.

3.3.4.7 Objections and Alternatives   Several objections can be raised against the proposed account of agrammatic comprehension. I will consider them in turn and then discuss alternative accounts. (Earlier objections and alternatives are addressed in Grodzinsky 1986a.)

The first objection concerns the fact that proposals such as the one made here can handle only three performance types: above-chance, at-chance, and below-chance. For this account, 80 percent accuracy (on a binary choice design) is virtually identical to 100 percent accuracy. Some might consider this a flaw, arguing that 80 percent accuracy is taken as evidence for an intact, normal-like representation, even though normal speakers *always* perform at 100 percent accuracy. Yet this type of criticism is unwarranted. If the agrammatic deficit is taken to be connected to either processing or the knowledge of grammatical principles, then, given that grammar is not defined probabilistically, distinctions that are finer than these three are irrelevant, and differences between, say, 80 percent and 90 percent accuracy are mere experimental artifacts. However, when discussing contrasts between above- and at-chance performance, some caution is necessary. In order to ensure that the distinctions sought are really found, it must be demonstrated that (1) the above-chance performance is significantly so, and (2) the two performances differ from one another significantly.

The second objection is that the agrammatic comprehension system violates principles of Universal Grammar. Specifically, given that the Theta Criterion constrains theta-role assignment and should ensure not only that the right number of roles is assigned but also that their identities match those listed on the theta-grid of the assigner, it can be argued that either agrammatic patients have lost the Theta Criterion or the account is incorrect. This issue has been considered by Sproat (1986), who cites independent evidence suggesting that knowledge of the Theta Criterion is preserved in agrammatism. Specifically, violations of this principle were easily detected by the patients tested by Linebarger, Schwartz, and Saffran (1983). Does that make the proposal incorrect, though? In my opinion, it does not. The representation that leads the patient to guessing is outside the linguistic system and therefore not subject to constraints like the Theta Criterion. The Default Principle that augments the patients' grammatical knowledge operates at a postgrammatical stage, and since their comprehension performance is aberrant with respect to theta-role assignment, it is not surprising that they exhibit some violations of the Theta Criterion. Nevertheless, we cannot conclude that they no longer know it. In fact, in chapter 5 we will see how this situation can motivate an argument for the modularity of the language processor.

The third objection concerns passive morphology. There is some evidence suggesting that, at least in some sense, the production deficit in agrammatism parallels the comprehension deficit. In particular, some investigators have argued that agrammatics are insensitive in comprehension to inflectional mor-phemes such as the passive one, precisely those that are omitted (or substituted for) in production. If this is so, then the agrammatic comprehension deficit might be accounted for by assuming that in interpreting passive sentences, the patients have access to the underspecified representation shown in (48).

(48) a. John$_i$ was [kill[ed] t_i] by Bill.
     b. John * kill* * by Bill.

Such a representation might simply create confusion on their part, and they would guess. The problem with this account is that it cannot be extended to either relative clauses or clefts, nor can it account for the consistent inversion of theta-roles seen with psychological verbs.

In addition, to say that by-phrases indicate agenthood in general (as suggested by Bates et al. (1986), for example) and that patients use them as cues to identify passive constructions is simply false, as can be seen from (49), where various nonagentive uses of by are demonstrated (see also Jaeggli 1986, section 4).

(49) a. The shell missed the tank by ten inches.
     b. He stood by the riverbank.
     c. John buys eggs by the dozen.
     d. The door was shut by the wind.
     e. Bill ruined his evening by going to a lousy movie.

To my knowledge, no data are available about the relative frequency of these uses. Hence, the claim that agrammatic patients use by as a cue for the agenthood of the following NP does not hold.

Similar arguments hold against proposals that capitalize on recent accounts of the passive, according to which the dethematization in passive constructions inheres in the absorption of the subject's theta-role by the passive morphology

(Jaeggli 1986) and its transmission to the oblique object. An account of agrammatism could be fashioned that would assume no such absorption and as a result would assume the subject of the passive to be a thematic position, assigned the role of agent, in conjunction with a *by*-phrase. Yet this account cannot be extended to other constructions that involve *wh*-traces.

A fourth objection concerns the analysis of passive assumed here. Specifically, there are reasons to believe that the *by*-phrase in verbal passives is governed. This is because it arguably does not fall under Huang's (1982) Condition on Extraction Domains, which states that extractions are possible from governed domains only. Consider (50), for example.

(50) a. Who was John [interested in *t*]?
    b. Who was John [pushed *t*] by *t'*?   (who is coindexed with *t'*)

In addition, if the passive *by* is assumed to be just a Case assigner and is assigned a theta-role by the passive morphology, then this assignment must take place under government. Under these assumptions, then, government does not account for the observed distinction between impaired and preserved prepositions.

There is, however, an alternative solution that captures the data accurately. Specifically, this solution locates the relevant difference in the identity of the theta-role assigner. Assume, following Jaeggli (1986) and Baker, Johnson, and Roberts (1989), that theta-role absorption in passives that involve movement is interpreted as assignment of the external theta-role to the passive morpheme *-en*, which in turn transmits it, under government, to the preposition *by*, if it is present. We now have two kinds of prepositional objects: those whose theta-role is directly assigned by the predicate (51a–b) and those whose theta-role is not (51c–d).

(51) a. John relied on Bill.
    b. John was interested in Bill.
    c. John was pushed by Bill.
    d. John sat on a chair.

These cases are partitioned correctly: agrammatic sensitivity to violations of grammaticality will be observed in cases where the prepositional object's theta-role is assigned by the predicate. We can thus easily replace the notion that the distinguishing criterion is government with the notion that it is the identity of the element that assigns the preposition its theta-role. Again, the theory naturally accounts for the data.

One could argue (as Lyn Frazier has suggested) that patients guess whenever the stimulus sentence deviates from the canonical order of constituents. Namely, in active, subject-relative, and subject-cleft sentences the NPs are ordered canonically around the verb, and in the other constructions under discussion they are not. Since agrammatics have no syntactic ability but can still deal with canonical arrangements, they do well on canonically ordered sentences, yet they guess whenever presented with a sentence that deviates from this order. The experimental result obtained with passive sentences containing psychological verbs (consistent inversion of theta-roles) shows that this possibility is unlikely, because it demonstrates that the aberrant behavior has a source other than simply order.

Another alternative is to argue that agrammatic patients have difficulties in handling complex linguistic material. This has often suggested, most recently by Goodglass and Menn (1985), who claim that "the comprehension of grammatical morphemes is involved in sentence comprehension only as a function of the cognitive difficulty of the relationship between lexical terms, which is signalled by the grammatical morphemes" (p. 22). An extension of this claim concerning perceptual complexity immediately comes to mind, namely, that the harder a construction is for a normal speaker to understand, the more likely it is that the agrammatic patient will fail to understand it. Yet this suggestion predicts a *gradation* in agrammatic comprehension, which is not found. Rather, the relevant studies reveal sharp drops from above-chance to at-chance to below-chance levels of performance (for discussion, see Grodzinsky, 1989).

Finally, it has been objected that the proposed account of agrammatic comprehension is not compelling because of the ad hoc status of the default strategy. Specifically, it is objected that since there is no general theory of strategies from which the particular one I propose would follow, it is hard to evaluate the account altogether. If another account were proposed, using a different strategy, the lack of a general theory of strategies would deprive us of the ability to decide between the two. (This has been suggested by Hagit Borer.) Although this point is true in principle, I am aware of no alternative account that is as parsimonious and descriptively adequate as mine. Moreover, the strategy I have proposed is quite plausible, and since our main interest here is not in developing a general theory of strategies, this will suffice.

3.3.4.8 Consequences and Predictions   Like any theoretically based descriptive statement, the one developed here is underdetermined by the data. It makes many untested predictions, some of which can actually resolve questions that it leaves open.

The predictions that follow most directly from the proposed descriptive generalization have to do with other constructions involving movement—in particular, constructions containing NP- or *wh*-traces. In every case the proposed account should predict whether performance is above, below, or at chance. I will not go into the details, because the interpretation of results may be problematic in some cases. Rather, I will restrict myself to giving examples of the relevant syntactic constructions. In English these include Raising sentences (52a–c) and questions (52e–h). In addition, short (agentless) passives (52d) should be tested, because they are predicted to yield below-chance performance, given that no grammatically assigned agent is present.[22]

(52) a. John seems [*t* to like Mary].
    b. John is believed [*t* to have left Mary].
    c. John appears [*t* crazy].
    d. John was shot *t*.
    e. Who [*t* shot John]?
    f. Who [did John shoot *t*]?
    g. [Which man] [*t* shot John]?
    h. [Which man] [did John shoot *t*]?

Other constructions—in fact, quite a few of them—also contain traces. An example from English is extraposition, illustrated in (53a–d). These sentences exemplify the interaction of two kinds of relations: extraposed/not-extraposed versus object/subject.

(53) a. A man *t* arrived [who *t* deserted a woman].
    b. A man *t* arrived [who a woman deserted *t*].
    c. A man [who *t* deserted a woman] arrived.
    d. A man [who a woman deserted *t*] arrived.

The next constructions involve other empty categories, of which there are four types: trace of NP-Movement, variable (a result of *Wh*-Movement at S-structure or of movement at the level of Logical Form), PRO (subject of infinitives and potentially noun phrases), and pro (in null-subject languages). (See Chomsky 1981, 1986a; Van Riemsdijk and Williams 1986; Bouchard 1984.) Each of these is constrained by different grammatical principles. PRO, for instance, is under the jurisdiction of control theory. Testing the behavior of aphasics on these can both refine the description of agrammatism and determine the status of these categories. For instance, the account I propose is limited to traces at S-structure. However, if it turns out that agrammatics err on PRO (as in (54)), or pro (as in the Hebrew example in (55)), then the conclusion will be that the notion "trace" has to be generalized to "empty category."

(54) a. John wanted [PRO to go].   (local control)
    b. It is time [PRO to go].   (arbitrary control)
    c. John told Mary about being obliged [PRO to go].(long-distance control)

(55) a. pro axalti banana
     pro ate-I   banana

   b. pro shamati she pro axalta banana
      pro heard-I that pro ate-you banana

If, on the other hand, it turns out that cases involving Quantifier Raising at the level of Logical Form (56) (May 1977, 1985) yield errors, then the notion "S-structure" in the description of agrammatism might have to be generalized, as well.

(56) a. Mary likes everyone.

   b. everyone [Mary likes t] (Logical Form)

It is not always clear how to test these constructions, because they do not all lend themselves to the experimental procedures that enable a straightforward interpretation. But if adequate methods are devised, it seems that all these empirical questions can be answered and that the description of agrammatism will have to be revised and modified.

There are yet other empty categories, whose status is a subject of debate. Examples of the latter category are the parasitic gaps, illustrated in (57) (see Engdahl 1980; Taraldsen 1979). It is not clear whether these are base-generated or traces of movement. Whatever the right description of agrammatism eventually turns out to be, it seems that the way these categories pattern might help in determining their theoretical status.

(57) a. Which books did you file t without reading t?

   b. He is a man who friends of t like t.

So far I have reviewed the predictions that the proposed account of agrammatism makes for constructions that contain empty categories. Yet there is reason to believe that future formulations will refer to coindexed categories rather than empty ones. That is, from the available evidence it is not at all clear whether the account should focus on the deleted category or on its link to an antecedent. To determine this issue, it will be necessary to test constructions that involve coindexing, but not empty elements—namely, anaphoric structures. There is a huge number of such constructions, and the particular choice will depend on the specific question being asked. Here we will briefly consider some arbitrarily selected examples, looking first at anaphors (58) and resumptive pronouns (59). (59a) and (59b) in fact constitute an especially interesting case, provided by Hebrew. Relative clauses that are derived by a transformation (59a) can also contain base-generated resumptive pronouns (59b), in whose derivation no transformations are involved (see Chomsky 1977).

(58) a. John likes himself.
    b. His mother likes John.
    c. John and Bill hate each other.

(59) a. ha-'ish she-ha-yalda ohevet hu tipesh
       the man that the girl loves is stupid
    b. ha-'ish she-ha-yalda ohevet oto   hu tipesh
       the man that the girl loves HIM is stupid

Other examples include violations of the Binding Conditions. If the impairment is not restricted to traces but instead extends to all cases of binding, then one prediction is that agrammatics will not be able to detect violations of Binding Condition C ("R-expressions must be free"). Even if they are aware of this condition, they might not have bound them, so no violation would follow. Consequently, they might err in judging the grammaticality of sentences like those in (60). (See chapter 4 for relevant preliminary results.)

(60) a. John likes John.
    b. John told Bill that he liked John.

Yet another interesting prediction concerns passive psychological verbs of the object-experiencer variety. These may have two readings, depending upon the PP complement they have. In (61a) a *by*-phrase forces a verbal reading of the sentence; hence, syntactic movement is implicated. In (61b), however, the adjectival reading indicates that the structure is base-generated with a PP complement (see Levin and Rappaport 1986).

(61) a. John was amused *t* by his colleagues.
    b. John was amused at his colleagues.

All these examples are but drops in the vast sea of structures for which a clear prediction follows from the proposed account. The facts, however, remain to be found.

A final issue concerns performance patterns across languages. In the discussion of speech production we have already seen how differences between languages correlate with differences in the performance patterns of agrammatic speakers of these languages. In comprehension, too, this correlation should hold even though hardly any evidence is available on this point.

The crucial parameter determining cross-linguistic differences from the present perspective is the nature of syntactic movement in a given language. We have seen that performance level on English structures containing traces of movement is determined by whether or not the moved NP crossed the verb. If it did—that is, if it moved from object to subject (in passive constructions) or to

Comp (in object-gap relative clauses)—then the default strategy assigns it an incorrect role, resulting in error. Otherwise (in subject-gap relatives and subject clefts), the strategy assigns a role that parallels the one the grammar should have assigned to that NP—cases of overlap, where the strategy compensates correctly for the agrammatic loss.

Having said that for English, one might now attempt to generalize to other configurational languages and predict the agrammatic performance as a function of syntactic properties of constructions. However, since the Default Principle is predicated on statistical regularities in large texts, it may have to be reformulated. Every cross-linguistic evaluation of the proposed account must therefore take into consideration both the properties of syntactic movement in a language and the nature of possible strategies used by its speakers. Keeping the strategy constant for the moment and concentrating on SVO languages, we can identify, in general, three relevant types of movement. In the first type (62a) an NP does not cross the verb or any other major (subject or object) NP in the sentence, in the second (62b) it crosses the verb only, and in the third (62c) one NP crosses another.

(62) a. . . .NP$_i$. .V. . .NP$_i$. . .

 b. . . .NP$_i$. . .V. . .NP$_i$

 c. . . .V. . .NP$_i$. . .NP$_i$. . .

Assuming that the strategy is like the one for English, then it should compensate correctly for (62a) and incorrectly for the rest.

3.4 Theoretical Issues

3.4.1 The Formal Status of the Characterization

I have proposed several modifications of the linguistic model, to capture generalizations concerning agrammatism. It is now time to examine the proposal from a formal point of view. Exactly what is the formal status of the deleted (or underspecified) elements? Or, to put the question another way, is the operation of deleting terminal elements from a representation consistent with the formal properties of the theory of grammar?

First, it is noteworthy that at least one formal theory of transformational grammar (Lasnik and Kupin 1977) cannot accommodate grammatical representations from which terminal elements have been deleted. Specifically, every nonterminal node must be expanded up to a terminal. This creates a potential problem. We could actually ignore this problem, arguing that the formal properties of the agrammatic language need not respect the constraints that the formalism imposes on normal grammar.[23] Yet should we choose to solve the problem, we can take one of two approaches. First, we could declare that whenever a terminal element is deleted, the branch dominating it is concomitantly pruned up to a branching node at S-structure. This will make (63a) look like (63b).

(63)

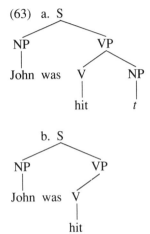

Yet such a proposal violates the Projection Principle, according to which lexical requirements (subcategorization) must be met at every level of representation. We are thus left with the second option, which does allow formal requirements to be met—namely, replacing every deleted category with a dummy symbol.

Another formal issue concerns the nature of the deleted elements. Consider the data in (64) (from Bouchard 1984), concerning the participation of empty categories in agreement.

(64) a. Anne seems [*t* to have hurt herself/*himself].   (NP-trace)
      b. Lisa tried [PRO to hide herself/*himself] behind the door.   (PRO)
      c. Which men did you say [*t* [*t* were/*was at the door]]?   (wh-trace)

Bouchard takes these facts to indicate that a part of the "content" of empty categories consists of tense and agreement features ("F-features" in his terminology). If these features are lexicalized at the level of Phonological Form, we have a lexical NP; if not, they are open to interpretation at the level of Logical Form. Traces thus contain F-features, as well as a referential index, linking them to their antecedent.

Now suppose that what happens in the agrammatic comprehension impairment is that a trace is deleted from S-structure representation along with its referential index. Following Bouchard's assumptions, we would expect that patients would have problems not only with theta-roles if traces are involved but also with agreement whenever it is mediated by a trace. It is known that agrammatic patients have problems with agreement in comprehension. We can thus derive an account of at least some of these problems directly from the Trace-Deletion Hypothesis: whenever agreement is mediated by a trace, it will be disrupted in agrammatism. This proposal leaves the rest of the agreement errors unexplained, however.

3.4.2 The Ontological Status of the Characterization

I have offered a description of pathological phenomena associated with one kind of brain damage. This account is not an independent *theory* of agrammatism. Rather, it is a descriptive generalization that captures given data in an economical way, while capitalizing on a conceptual framework provided by a well-motivated theory of syntactic representation. This description is formulated in order to *constrain* theoretical proposals concerning the mechanisms and knowledge base necessary for normal linguistic behavior. The manner in which these constraints function is described in the chapters that follow.

3.5 Conclusion

In this chapter I presented the data from agrammatic production and comprehension in such a way as to illustrate the existence of clear patterns, stated a generalization that accounts for cross-linguistic production data, and analyzed the results of several comprehension experiments according to performance level. I then showed how a minimal set of assumptions—some of them naturally couched in a theory of language structure, others in a theory concerning general cognitive resources—accounts for a whole range of pathological behaviors in agrammatic aphasia. On this basis, I propose a formal, theoretically motivated description of the syntactic disorder in agrammatism shown in (65).

(65) a. The S-structure representation underlying agrammatic speech production differs from the representation underlying normal speech production in the following respects:

    (i) Nonlexical terminals are deleted.

    (ii) Governed prepositions are deleted.

  b. The S-structure representation underlying agrammatic comprehension lacks traces. In interpretation, a Default Principle is invoked that is defined as follows:

If a lexical NP has no theta-role (that is, it is in a nonthematic position), assign it the theta-role that is canonically associated with the position it occupies, *unless* this assignment is blocked. In this case assign it a role from the next lower level in the Thematic Hierarchy.

This description is general; and although it will interact with the particulars of the language and syntactic construction in question, it is expected to give correct results. It does not mean, of course, that different knowledge systems underlie production and comprehension. Given that the descriptions of the agrammatic production and comprehension patterns cannot be collapsed, we are forced to claim that the two deficits are not parallel. This suggests (though it does not require) that the impairment affects the processing components, which differ in the two modalities.

Chapter 4
Neurological Constraints on Linguistic Theories

4.1 Introduction

In the past decade or so there has been a lot of brouhaha in cognitive science over the so-called psychological reality of theories of grammatical representation. Some linguists have attempted to motivate structural claims by referring to experimental data from the time-course of language comprehension (Bresnan 1978); others have relied on psychological metrics of complexity (Gazdar 1981). Psychologists, on the other hand, have continued their pursuit of evidence that would determine the "psychologically real" theory of language structure (Frazier, Clifton, and Randall 1983; Freedman and Forster 1985; Crain and Fodor 1985). These efforts can be interpreted in two ways: either as attempts to extend the domain of explanation of linguistic theory or as a search for external constraints on theories of grammar. And although the conceptual difference between these two approaches is minimal, I will adhere to the distinction for ease of exposition.

Here I should note parenthetically that the concept "psychological reality of grammars" does not always have a clear interpretation, and as a result many experiments stop short of providing a crucial test of it. In what follows I will attempt a new, different approach. I will confront neuropsychological evidence from aphasia—previously not taken into account by syntacticians—with syntactic theory. In fact, I will view data from agrammatic comprehension (and more specifically, the generalization over those data) as imposing a constraint on theories of language structure. Formulating my claim this way, I hope to avoid the pitfalls that have waylaid previous attempts.

The first view of the relation between experimental findings and linguistic theory is based on the assertion that although the standard object of explanation for linguistic theories is the grammatical intuitions of native speakers, these do not constitute the only available source of evidence about the language faculty.[1]

Facts about grammaticality, synonymy, and ambiguity help reveal crucial aspects of our linguistic ability, but there is other, less readily available evidence, obtained through psychological experiments. There is no reason, the argument runs, why this type of data should not be brought to bear on theories of language structure. After all, with the exception of some Platonists (see Katz 1981; Bever 1982), generative linguists have traditionally considered their field to be a branch of psychology, and the theory of syntax to be about the human linguistic capacity. Consequently, statements about regularities observed across sentences are taken to be statements about the structure of the human language faculty. In fact, the data linguistic theory normally uses are obtained via psychological experimentation, broadly construed: asking people about their linguistic intuitions is a psychological experiment par excellence. If this is the case, then any experimental piece of data might be of interest for linguists and should be in the domain of explanation of their theories.

In fact, the domain of explanation of syntactic theory has been extended over the years. Initially (for example, Chomsky 1957, 1965), generative grammarians sought an explanation for phenomena observed in one language (although in principle the intention was broader, of course). Later, they proposed extensions to account for language variation (such as Perlmutter's account of null subjects in Spanish, Rizzi's account of Subjacency in Italian, and Kayne's treatment of French), leading to the current "principles and parameters" approach. The approach under discussion aims at extending the data base in yet another direction—to include facts obtained by so-called psychological experiments, namely, data about linguistic aberrations (in development and breakdown), as well as the time-course of language processing.

The other view on the relevance of psychological experiments to linguistic theory is quite familiar. Linguists have always sought external sources to constrain their theoretical proposals, according to the principle that when a grammar obeys such constraints, its plausibility as a realistic theory of linguistic knowledge is greatly increased. Specifically, they have required that their theory be *learnable* and *parsable*. Chomsky (1955), for instance, proposes the *learnability* criterion to constrain the set of possible grammars for a language. He suggests that among the many grammars that are found to describe English adequately, the one that should be chosen as the "correct" theory is the one that is most easily learnable (in his case the one with the smallest number of symbols), so as to account for the ease and regularity with which humans attain their linguistic capacity. The learnability criterion is thus external in that it is not in the domain of linguistic theory, its establishment justifies the theory, and it actually serves as a theoretical constraint: only learnable grammars are to be considered seriously as theories of linguistic knowledge. Indeed, some have argued that versions of generative grammar meet the learnability constraint (Pinker 1982; Wexler and Culicover 1980).

A second external criterion that is commonly proposed is *parsability*. (See Miller and Chomsky 1963. For more recent discussion, see Berwick and Weinberg 1984; Fodor 1985; Culicover 1985.) If a grammar is a theory of our knowledge of language L, and if this knowledge is brought to use efficiently, as seems to be the case—that is, if we are able to analyze the structure of incoming strings of L on-line—then our grammar must have associated with it an algorithm that guarantees that any string in L can be parsed correctly in nonexponential time. Moreover, the algorithm must carry out this task in the way that humans actually do.

These two constraints are concerned with the biological feasibility of linguistic theory. In the present context this immediately suggests a third constraint that should be imposed on linguistic theory: it must be neurologically adequate. This can be guaranteed if there is evidence that whenever some language-relevant function breaks down along structural lines, the pattern of loss and sparing is compatible with whatever postulates the theory dictates. That is, in a selective loss of linguistic capacities it should always be the case that the patterns of loss and sparing form natural classes in the theory. We can thus require our theory to meet the criterion of *breakdown-compatibility:* every pattern of impairment and sparing of linguistic ability must be accounted for in a natural, non–ad hoc fashion. This requirement is not unqualified; later we will consider its precise nature and the conditions under which it applies.

The recent psycholinguistic studies mentioned earlier are certainly not the first attempts to provide evidence for or against the "psychological reality" of one theory or another. Indeed, in the last twenty-five years many psychological considerations and experimental findings have been claimed to provide such evidence, among them the reaction-time experiments done in the 1960s in the framework of the Derivational Theory of Complexity (see Fodor, Bever, and Garrett 1974 for an excellent review) and the experimentally based claims advanced in the 1970s concerning the so-called autonomy of syntax (see Marslen-Wilson and Tyler 1980). In general, however, it can be said that such claims, based always on analyses of the time-course of language comprehension, have been largely ignored in generative circles. Many were seen as insufficiently detailed to warrant serious consideration, and some were simply beside the point, or involved problematic assumptions, or provided evidence that was far from compelling. The argument that linguistic theory is accountable to the data generated experimentally was countered with the argument that until a well-articulated theory of complexity and of the time-course of language processing becomes available, the mapping between knowledge structures and the processes that implement them is far from clear.

This chapter, then, is about the linguistic relevance of deficit analyses of aphasic syndromes. Although the discussion will focus on language deficits and linguistic theories, the form of the argument should in principle be generalizable to any cognitive domain, defined by a theory, in which selective deficits are observed.

The argument will proceed along these lines. Suppose that an insult to some area of the brain results in selective loss of the ability to understand and produce sentences. The nature of the functional deficit depends on the anatomical site of the damage, which in turn is determined by the distribution of cerebral blood vessels, one or more of which has been ruptured or clogged, causing the brain damage. To be sure, it is hardly imaginable that these physical variables will play an explanatory role in an abstract theory of language structure. From the point of view of this theory, the anatomical facts are completely arbitrary. Indeed, most language disturbances seem to have very little to do with knowledge of language. Rather, they affect specific modalities for use in ways that are uninteresting from the present perspective (Goodglass and Kaplan 1972; Geschwind 1979).

The situation changes, however, if we encounter a loss that can be shown to be selective from a structural point of view. If we can find a case in which the brain-damaged patient is able to understand sentences of some syntactic types but not others, this will be of potential interest for the theory of syntax. What we might have in this case is selective impairment to language mechanisms, where the selectivity is governed by structural principles. If such a case can indeed be found, it might serve as a powerful test for the biological feasibility of specific theoretical models in the following way: if a part of the language faculty is lost, and if our theory of structure is about this faculty, then the characterization of the structural deficit following this loss must be accommodated in the theory in a natural way. In other words, the theory must be able to state generalizations over the patterns of loss and sparing following brain damage. If it meets this requirement, it is breakdown-compatible. So, although there does not seem to be a necessary match between some arbitrary damage to a cortical site and the theory of syntax, it should now be apparent why there may be language deficits that are directly relevant to linguistics. We can use data from selective brain damage (aphasic syndromes) to motivate neurologically based constraints on linguistic theory. Consequently, these constraints can help us evaluate grammatical frameworks, by obliging them to meet the requirement of breakdown-compatibility. A theory that meets this requirement will be taken to be more highly constrained than a theory that does not.

There may be many instances of the breakdown-compatibility constraint, depending on observable patterns of erroneous performance caused by physical damage to the language faculty. Naturally, the more cases that are discovered, the more highly constrained the theory of grammar will be, from a neuropsychological point of view. In the following section I will state one such constraint on linguistic theories, based on the description of agrammatism proposed in chapter 3, and I will evaluate various theories of syntactic representation according to that constraint. First, however, I would like to consider another preliminary issue: the source of the impairment and its relevance to my argument.

As we have seen, there are two possible causes for the observed functional deficit in aphasia: it could result either from a loss of grammatical knowledge per se (whereby the patient no longer "knows" some aspects of grammar) or from a disruption to some process(es) that put knowledge to use. Indeed, in chapter 3 I did not decide between these possibilities. This makes little difference for the present argument, however. Suppose the grammatical knowledge base is impaired. Then the way it is impaired is obviously relevant to the theory of syntax: the theory, which is about human grammatical knowledge, must be compatible with the observed deficit, since this deficit reflects the internal organization of grammatical knowledge. This compatibility is ensured just in case the pattern of impairment forms a natural class within the theory. If the impairment resulted from a knowledge deficit, then, the theory would be breakdown-compatible if the distinctions that the brain makes, as evidenced by breakdown patterns, could be stated in the theory in a natural way. On the other hand, the loss could result from a processing disruption. In this case the same argument still holds if the relation between the grammar and the algorithms putting it to use is taken to be other than arbitrary. That is, the processes involved in recovering grammatical structure in the course of interpretation must make distinctions that are similar to those made by the grammar. In this case disruption to a processor that is responsible for recovering structures dictated by a particular linguistic theory will still have to meet the breakdown-compatibility requirement. The formal description of agrammatism is therefore of potential interest in the present context, whatever the precise nature of the antecedent impairment is.

We thus have a general method for evaluating linguistic theories against data from aphasia: First find out whether the pattern of loss is structural. If it is, state a descriptive generalization over it, derive its consequences, and test them. Finally, determine whether this description can be stated in the theory. Linguistic theory is thus accountable for patterns of breakdown and sparing following brain damage.

Having clarified these methodological questions, I will use the suggested method to present my argument concerning the breakdown-compatibility of current syntactic theories. I will discuss two instances where the constraints can be applied. First, I will compare three syntactic frameworks in light of the formal description of agrammatic comprehension (specifically, comprehension of the passive construction), concluding that the observed pattern is naturally described by Government-Binding Theory, yet it is virtually unstatable in the framework of Lexical-Functional Grammar (Bresnan 1982b) or Generalized Phrase Structure Grammar (Gazdar et al. 1985). Ad hoc machinery needs to be stipulated in order for these theories to account for the data. I will claim that the breakdown-compatibility constraint is therefore met only by GB Theory, and I will take this as evidence in support of this class of theories, and against the others.[2]

As a second case, I will discuss an internal debate within the GB theoretical framework. I will evaluate two proposed formulations of the Binding Conditions (Chomsky 1981; Reinhart 1983) in light of experimental findings from aphasia (Grodzinsky et al. 1989). Here, too, I will argue that only one formulation—the one proposed by Reinhart—meets the breakdown compatibility constraint.

4.2   A Neurological Constraint: The Analysis of Passive

4.2.1   The Lexical-Transformational Controversy concerning Passive
The analysis of the passive construction has been at the center of a major theoretical debate in generative linguistics. Some theoretical frameworks conceive of passivization as a lexical process (Bresnan 1982a; Gazdar et al. 1985), whereas others view certain passives as lexical and others as derived transformationally (Chomsky 1981). The following section presents the essentials of the different analyses and then discusses them in light of the description of agrammatic comprehension.

4.2.2   A Government-Binding Account of Verbal and Adjectival Passives
It is generally held in GB accounts that there are two types of passive participles in English, syntactically derived verbal passive and lexically derived adjectival passive . Both are analyzed as undergoing a preliminary lexical process, the attachment of the verbal suffix. This morphological change affects the inherent Case-assigning properties of the verb. With respect to verbal passive, suppression of the external theta-role and accusative Case, either via absorption (Chomsky 1981) or via assignment to the passive morpheme (Jaeggli 1986), leads to NP-movement of the thematic object to subject position, resulting in a trace in [NP,VP] position. In adjectival passive formation, on the other hand, further lexical processes result in the elimination of the [NP,VP] position and the

externalization of the internal theta-role. In other words, the adjectival passive participle is constrained to be predicated of the direct object of the root verb (Levin and Rappaport 1986). No movement occurs and no traces arise.

The two passive formation processes are clearly similar. One important difference, for our purposes, is that only syntactic passive formation produces a structure containing an NP-trace. Although the internal theta-role is externalized in the process of lexical affixation, it is not affected in the syntactic process. This means that the internal theta-role is assigned in the normal fashion to direct object position. But because accusative Case is no longer available for assignment to that position, the object NP moves to subject position, leaving a coindexed trace behind. An example is given in (1).

(1)   a.   D-structure: *e* was kicked the ball
      b.   S-structure: [The ball]$_i$ was kicked [e_i]

Another crucial difference concerns the subject theta-role. In lexical passivization, the external theta-role is eliminated. In syntactic passivization, the external theta-role is preserved. That is, it is assigned to the passive morpheme, from where it is optionally transmitted to the object of *by* in the full passive (Baker, Johnson, and Roberts 1989). Instances of thematic (nonargument) control into embedded purpose clauses serve as evidence that an agent is in fact syntactically present in the truncated verbal passive.

(2)   a.   The ball was kicked [PRO to get the game going].
      b.   The park was destroyed [PRO to construct new housing].

PRO in these embedded clauses is subject to thematic control by the implicit agent of a passivized verb.

Despite these differences, the distinction between the two passives is far from clear-cut. Many participles distribute in both adjectival and verbal contexts, as can be seen from (3).

(3)   a.   Mary was [$_{AP}$highly impressed].
      b.   Mary$_i$ was [$_{VP}$impressed e_i by John].

Although there are many verbal passives that do not distribute as adjectives (for example, *the killed woman, *the seen painting*), the majority of adjectival passives are homophonous with verbal passives. That is, they may also be derived syntactically. The structure in (3a) is in fact ambiguous between verbal and adjectival interpretations. The *by*-phrase in (3b), however, can be said to force a transitive reading of the participle.

Some verbs, including a subset of the class of psychological verbs, occur more frequently in the passive than in the active (for instance, *pleased, amused, interested*). Use of the *by*-phrase with these participles is somewhat awkward. Other prepositions, including *with, in,* and *about,* normally head source phrases in these constructions, as illustrated in (4).

(4)   a. Mary was concerned about John.
      b. ?Mary was concerned by John.

Because of the contrast in (4), and also because use of a by-phrase forces the transitive reading, all items implemented in the Adjectival Passive Condition of our experiment do not occur with *by*-phrases.

The only productive, nonidiosyncratic subclass of adjectival passives of the strictly lexical type are those adjectival passives that undergo additional morpheme affixation. Certain morphemes, including *semi, much,* and (most commonly), negative *un,* prefix to adjectives (*much-loved, unhappy, unconvinced*) but never to verbs (**unkill, *unthrow*). Negative *un* is thus not to be confused with reversative *un,* which attaches only to verbs and indicates the reversal of an action (*uncap, undress*).

Unlike other adjectives with passive morphology, the so-called *un*-passives distribute more freely with *by*-phrases.

(5)   a. i.?John was interested by Mary.
         ii.*John was devoted by Mary.
      b. i. John was interested in Mary.
         ii. John was devoted to Mary.
      c. i. John was unloved by Mary.
         ii. John was unnoticed by Mary.
      d. i.*Mary unloved John.
         ii.*Mary unnoticed John.

Given the unacceptability of (5d), however, it can be argued that *un* in (5c) has scope over the whole of the participial phrase. We will return to these and other aspects of the *un*-passive in the sections below.

4.2.3   LFG Analysis

Lexical Functional Grammar (LFG) maintains that all passives are lexical. In order to account for the differences between adjectival and verbal passives, it assumes two types of lexical rules for passives. The rule for verbal passives changes grammatical functions (which are taken to be primitives in this theory), generating representations such as (5). Adjectival passives are derived from these forms (6), which also has an output condition, as can be seen in (5)–(6) ((3) and (36) in Bresnan 1982a).

(5) Mary hit John.   John was hit (by Mary).
     | | | |
     SUBJ   OBJ   SUBJ   (OBJ)

     Functional change: SUBJ $\rightarrow$ O/(BY OBJ)
                              OBJ $\rightarrow$ SUBJ

     Morphological change: V $\rightarrow$ V$_{Part}$

(6) a. The dog was eaten.
     b. the eaten dog

     Morphological change: V$_{Part}$ $\rightarrow$ [V$_{Part\ A}$]
     Operation on lexical form:
                    P(...(SUBJ)...) $\rightarrow$ STATE-OF P(...(SUBJ)...)
                    Condition: SUBJ = theme of P

Importantly, we can see that the lexical operations that apply in the derivation of passives (whether verbal or adjectival) are not the same kind that apply in the derivation of questions, relative clauses, clefts, and other long-distance dependencies. This fact is crucial for the argument I present later.

4.2.4 Generalized Phrase Structure Analysis

As in LFG, the passive in Generalized Phrase Structure Grammar (GPSG) is not derived by a transformation. Unlike what happens in LFG, however, the relation between actives and passives is captured in GPSG by a statement relating not to categories but *rules* of grammar—in this case phrase structure rules that generate actives with those that generate passives. GPSG posits several such generalizations, called *metarules*. The general format for metarules is stated in (7a) and the passive metarule in (7b): (from Gazdar et al. 1985).

(7) a. $a_0 \rightarrow a_1, \ldots, a_n$
                    $\Downarrow$
         $b_0 \rightarrow b\text{-}[1], \ldots, b_n$

     b. VP $\rightarrow$ W,NP
                    $\Downarrow$
         VP[PAS] $\rightarrow$ W, (PP[*by*])

This rule is interpreted as follows: for every rule in the grammar in which a VP immediately dominates an NP and some other material W, there is also a rule that permits the passive category VP[PAS] to dominate just the other material from the original rule, together (optionally) with a PP containing a *by*-phrase.

Crucially, as in LFG, long-distance dependencies are subject to completely different generalizations in GPSG, being generated by other mechanisms.

4.2.5   A Crucial Test Case from Agrammatism

In chapter 3 I assumed uncritically the GB Theory analysis of passive. Now it is time to question this assumption, which is reflected, of course, in the descriptive statement I proposed for agrammatic comprehension patterns.

(8)   The S-structure representation underlying agrammatic comprehension lacks traces. In interpretation, a Default Principle is invoked that is defined as follows:

If a lexical NP has no theta-role (that is, it is in a nonthematic position), assign it the theta-role that is canonically associated with the position it occupies, unless this assignment is blocked. In this case assign it a role from the next lower level in the Thematic Hierarchy.

If we take the analyses of passive that the three theories maintain, in conjunction with other grammatical principles, we find that so far all three systems can account for the data, with varying degrees of elegance. The GB Theory account has been presented. The LFG account would presumably state that the patient's grammatical system represents neither unbounded dependencies (for relatives) nor lexical relations (for passives).[3] GPSG would state a disruption to mechanisms responsible for unbounded dependencies and would presumably block the passive metarule. More data are necessary to distinguish the three theories. A crucial test, it seems, lies in the case of adjectival (lexical) passives.

Consider the various rule types in each of the theories and how their domains differ. In GB Theory, questions, relatives, and verbal passives are transformationally derived; lexical passives and other lexically derived forms, such as *un-*passives and *-able* adjectives, are derived by a lexical rule. In LFG and GPSG all passives are lexical, and questions and relatives are derived by an algorithm that links gaps to their antecedents.

(9)   Construction   GB   LFG-GPSG
      a. John was interested in Mary.   lexical   lexical
      b. John was kicked by Mary.   syntactic   lexical
      c. The man who Mary kicked was tall.   syntactic   syntactic

Given this contrast between the two classes of theories, and with the descriptive generalization over the agrammatic data in mind, the most obvious move is to look at adjectival passives. If these pattern with actives in contrast to the syntactic passives and object relatives, the GB account will still hold, since adjectival passives are derived by a lexical rule in this framework, and thus their representations do not contain a trace. An LFG account will not be possible in this case, since LFG cannot state a generalization over verbal passives and relatives, in contrast to lexical passives. If anything, LFG predicts that all passives will pattern together, in contrast to unbounded dependencies. In sum, then, the Trace-Deletion Hypothesis predicts that agrammatic patients should exhibit no comprehension problems when presented with adjectival passives, despite their apparent similarity to their verbal counterparts.

Amy Pierce and I (Grodzinsky and Pierce 1987) have designed and conducted an experiment to test these predictions. It entails six conditions, corresponding to the six sentence types shown in (10).

(10) a. Agentive actives: The man is pushing the boy.
    b. Un-reversative actives: The mother unmasks the girl
    c. Adjectival passives: The doctor was annoyed with the boy.
    d. Un-passives: The woman was uninspired by the man.
    e. Un-verbal passives: The girl is unmasked by the mother.
    f. Agentive passives: The boy is pushed by the man.[4]

Twenty sentences of each type were presented to patients in random order. In order to preserve the adjectival reading, adjectives with passive morphology were presented without by-phrases; *about-*, *with-*, *at-*, and *in*-phrases were used instead.

The results largely bear out the prediction of the account based on the mixed GB analysis of passives. Two agrammatic patients have been tested and were found to perform virtually identically. The results are shown in (11a–f)— corresponding to (10a–f), respectively—coded for percentage of sentences correctly interpreted.

(11) a. Agentive actives: 92.5%
    b. Un-reversative actives: 87.5%
    c. Adjectival passives: 82.5%
    d. Un-passives: 57.5%
    e. Un-verbal passives: 52.5%
    f. Agentive passives: 60.0%

The numbers reflect a clear-cut distinction: above-chance performance on conditions (a) through (c), and a sharp drop to chance-level performance on conditions (d) through (f). Thus, the patients performed well on both types of actives and on adjectives with passive morphology, as predicted by the GB-based account, and contrary to the prediction of lexical theory. Therefore, only the former is breakdown-compatible.

An unexpected result, however, is the chance-level performance on un-passives cooccurring with *by*-phrases, like those in (12).

(12) a. The man was unconvinced by the woman.

     b. The queen was unimpressed by the king.

There are four ways to interpret this outcome. First, patients might simply be insensitive to the *un* morpheme, as they are said to be to closed-class vocabulary in general, thereby interpreting (12a) as (13).

(13) The man (was) convinced (by) the woman.

This seems unlikely, however, since (1) patients do not report a mismatch between such sentences when presented with their pictorial representations, (2) results from the un-reversative active condition indicate no such omission of the *un* prefix, and (3) there is independent experimental evidence that agrammatics are sensitive to the preposition *by*.

Second, it has often been suggested that perhaps agrammatic patients' problem with syntactic passive can simply be attributed in its entirety to an insensitivity to passive morphology. Yet this analysis fails to account for the prior findings concerning object-gap relatives and clefts—the fact that agrammatics have difficulty with wh-constructions as well as with syntactic passive constructions.

Third, it may be that hypersensitivity to the *by*-phrase as a signal of passive voice forces a transitive reading of the un-passive verb. This analysis, however, falls short of explaining the relatively large number of errors made by normal control subjects on un-passives. The results from normal subjects suggest difficulty with the un-passive construction in general, a difficulty that perhaps is exacerbated in aphasia.

As a related possibility, we consider the explanation that *un*-passives are in fact syntactically derived. Poor performance would then follow from the deletion of the trace in the representation of the *un*-passive. Such an account proceeds as follows: We first assume that the two prefixes *un* (the reversative as in *untie* and the unpassive as in *uninhabited*) are in fact one and differ in their level of affixation. Although the reversative affix is lexical, the *un*-passive is a syntactic affix (see Fabb 1984), adjoined to VP with scope over the whole of the participial phrase. This accounts for the contrasts in (14).

(14) a.   John untied the prisoner.

     b. *The argument unconvinced Bill.

The fact that *un*-passives seem to pattern with adjectives in certain environments is thus accounted for by the properties of the affix. Although regular participles cannot be complements of raising verbs, *un*-passives, like adjectives, can. This analysis also accounts for the fact that *un*-passives do not have deverbal nouns, such as *unimpression*. If the affixation process were in the lexicon, then nothing would block their derivation. Similar considerations hold for derived nominals.

(15) a. Bill's unmasking by John
    b. *John's unconvincing by the argument

In addition, passives with *by*-phrases are only analyzable as being syntactically derived, as the *by*-phrase forces a transitive interpretation of the participle. Therefore, all passives with *by*-phrases contain traces in canonical direct object position.

Under these assumptions, an unpassive such as (12b) would then be analyzed as having the structure in (16).

(16) [The queen]$_i$ was [$_{VP}$un-[$_{VP}$impressed t_i by the king]].

According to this analysis, the *un*-passive with a *by*-phrase is a case of an adjectival passive that is syntactically derived.

To summarize, the proposal here is that the guessing performance of the agrammatic patients observed in the *Un*-passive Condition is potentially attributable to syntactic derivation. Due to affixation of the passive morpheme in syntax, unpassives with *by*-phrases contain traces at S-structure. As a result of their grammatical deficit, agrammatics delete these traces and, in the manner described, end up with an interpretation involving two NP agents between which they can only guess. At the very least, the results of this condition indicate that a reexamination of the *un*-passive along the lines sketched above is in order .

4.3 Agrammatism and Binding Theory: Another Test Case?

Some hints from aphasia are now available regarding another current debate in syntax, in connection with the formulation of the Binding Conditions. One approach (Chomsky 1981; see chapter 2) states separate Binding Conditions to govern the distribution of anaphors (A), pronouns (B), and names (C), whereas another (Reinhart 1983, 1986) dispenses with the need to state a special condition for names. In addition, Chomsky claims that reflexives and pronouns fall under different generalizations—Conditions A and B, respectively; Reinhart, on the other hand, contends that although reflexives are subject to Condition A, only certain pronouns (bound variables) fall under Condition B. For her, the significant generalization is an interpretive rule that is stated over anaphors and some of the pronouns, which are viewed as bound variables, whereas the interpretation of the rest of the pronouns (in cases of coreference) is determined by discourse. There is some evidence from language acquisition (Wexler and Chien 1988) suggesting that the latter view is correct—that bound variables (both pronouns and reflexives) are distinct from the rest of the pronouns in that their rates of acquisition are different. Some new data from aphasia lead to the same conclusion, thus strengthening the evidential basis of Reinhart's claim.

Since the motivation for the Binding Conditions was presented in chapter 2, the discussion here centers around Reinhart's proposal and the differences between the two approaches. Consider the Binding Conditions as proposed by Chomsky (1981):

(17) A. An anaphor must be bound in its governing category.
     B. A pronoun must be free in its governing category.
     C. An R-expression [name] must be free.

Condition A controls the distribution of anaphors and serves both to force coreference in sentences like *John washed himself* and to exclude ungrammatical cases like **John asked Mary to wash himself*. Condition B regulates pronouns, excluding cases like *John washed him*, where John and him corefer. Condition C handles cases in which names have local antecedents. It declares strings such as *He washed John*, where the name and the pronoun corefer, as ungrammatical.

Reinhart accepts Conditions A and B, but rejects C. Moreover, the scope of Condition B for her is limited to cases where the antecedent c-commands the pronoun. In such cases the pronoun is interpreted as a bound variable. The motivation for this change comes, initially, from facts about pronouns bound to quantified antecedents. These are subject to stronger structural conditions for binding. Observe the contrast in (18), where coreference between the pronouns and a name is possible in (18a) but ruled out in (18b).

(18) a. His father came with John.
     b. *His father came with each boy.

GB theorists account for this difference by assuming a special LF condition on quantifiers (the Bijection Principle) that rules out (18b) and similar cases. Yet Reinhart observes that pronouns can function as bound variables also in certain cases where the antecedent is an R-expression, thus outside the scope of the Bijection Principle. Some of these are illustrated in (19a–c).

(19) a. Max walked his dog and Charlie did, too.
        i. For X = Max, X walked X's dog, and for Y = Charlie, Y walked Y's dog.
        ii. For X = Max, X walked X's dog, and for Y = Charlie, Y walked X's dog.
     b. Only Max voted for his mother.
        i. For X = Max, only X voted for X's mother.
        ii. For X = Max, only X voted for Max's mother.

c. The attempt to assassinate the Pope scared him, and the Prime Minister too.

Each of these sentences is multiply ambiguous. (19a) can mean either that each person walked his own dog (i) or that both walked Max's dog (ii). (19b) can entail either that Max's mother may have gotten many votes, but among the mother-candidates she was the only one for whom her son voted (i), or that Max's mother indeed got one vote, Max's (ii). This ambiguity indicates that pronouns may be bound variables, yet sometimes they are not.

These facts (as well as methodological considerations) lead Reinhart to her proposal: a system that distinguishes between binding and coreference. Binding is the relation that holds between an anaphor or a pronoun and a c-commanding antecedent—a syntactic relation crucial for the interpretation of bound variables; coreference between pronouns that are not bound variables and their antecedents need not be represented in the syntax but can be handled by other considerations. Her theory accounts for Condition B effects in two ways: cases of coreference (or noncoreference) are handled by an inference rule; cases of pronouns that are bound variables (or restrictions against such readings) are handled by an interpretive rule. The same rule handles the effects of Condition C. Reinhart assumes free coindexing—a process that assigns an index to pronouns and antecedents—and an interpretive rule. The latter is of the form shown in (20).

(20) For any given node α, replace the index of α and all NPs that α binds at S-structure with an identical variable index.

The idea, then, is that the interpretive rule, not the coindexing procedure, is what excludes bound variable readings when they are impossible. That is, pronouns such as the one in (21b) cannot corefer with a local antecedent, not by virtue of Binding Condition B, but because they are incompatible with the interpretive rule (20).

(21) a. John read his book.
    For X = John, X read X's book.
    b. He read John's book.

In (21a) free coindexing makes the bound variable reading possible. In (21b), however, the pronoun does not have an antecedent and the interpretive rule therefore cannot assign a bound variable reading. Note that this reading is excluded without stating a special Binding Condition for names. Instead of claiming that (21b) is ruled out because the name cannot be bound—as Chomsky's Condition C would do—we are now claiming that it is ruled out because the pronoun is not bound.

What about coreference? After all, many constructions lacking a bound variable allow coreference. Look at (19c), for example. A "coreference" reading is possible, where both personalities were scared by the attempted assassination of the Pope, but the "bound variable" reading, where two assassination attempts were made (one on the Pope and one on the Prime Minister), is unavailable. According to Reinhart, all these facts indicate that we are dealing with two different issues here, and she proposes that coreference is governed by separate rules. This is problematic, however. If coreference is possible in (19c), then why is it impossible in (21b)? To solve this problem, Reinhart conditions the application of the inference rule on the satisfaction of a syntactic condition. Namely, coreference is allowed only if the pronoun in question is in a position of which binding could not hold. Thus, coreference is not allowed in (22a) because the speaker could use a reflexive (22b); the fact that the speaker chose not to indicates that coreference was not intended. (22c–d), on the other hand, demonstrate exactly the opposite: coreference is possible because binding is not.

(22) a. John washed him. (* on coreferential reading)
     b. John washed himself.
     c. *John asked Mary to wash himself.
     d. John asked Mary to wash him.

Opponents of this view—for instance, Higginbotham (1985)—argue that this principle does not work for cases like (23).

(23) a. They saw him.
     b. *They saw himself.
     c. John and Mary saw him.
     d. *John and Mary saw himself.

In these cases the pronoun cannot be replaced by a reflexive, and still noncoreference is required. This suggests to Higginbotham that Binding Condition B holds for all pronouns, whereas phenomena associated with quantified antecedents are actually distinguished at LF.

This cursory review leads to the following conclusions. First, Reinhart's generalization, but not Chomsky's, holds for the binding of both reflexives and bound pronouns, regardless of the quantificational properties of their antecedents. According to Reinhart's theory, they are all anaphors that fall under the interpretive rule. In GB studies of anaphora, however, pronouns with quantified NP antecedents must be bound variables because it makes no sense to talk about coreference with quantified NPs (like *each of the girls*) that have no reference themselves. Thus, the nature of the antecedent determines whether a pronoun will be a bound variable or will enter into a coreference relation. The former situation is handled by LF conditions. For reflexives, however, a bound variable reading must be forced (by Condition A). Notice, however, that the sentences in (19) contain definite NP antecedents, not quantifiers, and still a bound variable reading is allowed (19ai,bi). This is Reinhart's strongest argument in favor of her approach and against Chomsky's (see Reinhart 1986, 126).

Second, Chomsky, unlike Reinhart, handles coreference in a way that is independent of syntactic binding. According to Chomsky's theory, coreference is free, unless excluded by Condition B; according to Reinhart's, coreference is possible if and only if a syntactic condition (that has to do with anaphoric binding) is met. Third, Chomsky's theory, unlike Reinhart's, needs a special condition that prohibits the binding of names (Condition C).

Let us now turn to the experimental evidence that bears on this debate. In a test conducted with young children, Wexler and Chien (1988) showed that Reinhart's formulation is correct. On a comprehension task involving sentences and pictures, they found that young children could interpret reflexives and bound pronouns at a rather early stage of their linguistic development, yet their ability to comprehend coreference relations lagged behind. They took this finding to indicate that the correct generalization is along the lines suggested by Reinhart (see chapter 6 for elaboration).

Following this study, and acting on previous clues suggesting selective impairment in aphasia in this domain (Blumstein et al. 1983), several colleagues and I have explored the ability of agrammatic patients to comprehend pronouns and anaphors (Grodzinsky et al., 1989). The details of the experiment are presented in chapter 6; here I will review only the data that are directly relevant to the present discussion.

The stimuli in this experiment were sentences like the ones in (24) containing reflexives and pronouns with varied antecedents.

(24) a. Is Mama Bear washing herself?
   b. Is Mama Bear washing her?
   c. Is every bear washing her?

The patients in our experiment (like the children in Wexler and Chien's study) were supposed to give a yes/no answer when the sentence and a picture were presented to them. The pictures were of either reflexive actions (to match sentences like (24a)) or transitive actions (to match (24b–c)), and each sentence was presented with both a matching and a nonmatching picture. Other control conditions were also given, with 12 tokens each. The patients performed nearly perfectly on reflexives (24a) and at chance on (24b)—results that are strikingly similar to those Wexler and Chien found for children. The crucial condition, however, was (24c), containing a pronoun with a quantified NP antecedent. A quantifier in this position forces a bound variable reading, as illustrated in (25).

(25) Every boy walked his dog, and Steve did, too.
For every X, X = boy, X walked X's dog, and for Y = Steve,
Y walked Y's dog.

Crucially, the reading on which Steve walked every boy's dog, but not his own, is excluded, which shows (unsurprisingly) that the coreferential reading that is available in (19) is unavailable here, where a bound variable reading is forced. Definite NP antecedents allow both a bound variable reading and coreference, whereas quantified NP antecedents allow the former only. It follows that the contrast between (24b) and (24c) stems from the fact that in the former noncoreference is determined by discourse, whereas in the latter it is determined by the interpretive rule (20). Put differently, the knowledge that coreference is impossible in (24b) presupposes knowledge of the pragmatic conditions that govern the distribution of pronouns, but for (24c) both discourse and syntactic conditions may be used. Thus, the absence of pragmatic knowledge will lead to poor performance on (24b), yet on (24c) speakers can resort to syntactic knowledge, if it is at their disposal. All this is according to Reinhart.

The findings presented so far are compatible with both Reinhart's approach and the GB approach. Reinhart would say that rule (20) is available—explaining the patients' good performance in the "reflexive" condition (24a)—and the pragmatic principle is gone—explaining their poor performance in the "pronoun" condition (24b). The GB view would hold that Condition A is intact, whereas Condition B is not. Obviously, the crucial case is (24c), containing a pronoun with a quantified NP antecedent, because it falls under a different generalization in each theory.

The patients, it was found, performed above chance in this condition. The standard GB framework cannot readily account for this fact, yet Reinhart's system can. The GB approach would predict that condition (24c) would yield poor performance, because it falls under Binding Condition B. Reinhart's system, however, would say that because the bound variable reading is excluded on syntactic as well as pragmatic grounds, even though the patients have no access to pragmatic knowledge (as shown by their poor performance in the "pronoun" condition), they can still make use of their syntactic knowledge (attested in the "reflexive" condition) to exclude coreference in (24c) and perform correctly, as they did. Noam Chomsky (personal communication) suggests that the GB approach can account for the experimental results by saying that Condition B is stated as holding of bound pronouns, in conjunction with a dictum that it be regularized to all pronouns. According to this proposal, it is the second statement that children develop and aphasics lose. This proposal, however, raises certain questions. First, why would such a principle exist? Is there any other domain in syntax where knowledge of some part of grammar is there from the beginning stages, yet its domain is extended through language development? Second, why would the first developmental stage start with bound variables and extend itself, and not in another fashion? Third, why is the extension lost in aphasia? These questions do not arise if Reinhart's system is adopted. Thus, whether or not hers is the right formulation, there is no doubt that Condition B must be reformulated if it is to account for the aphasia and language acquisition data. In fact, this reformulation should be undertaken on the basis of data that could not be obtained by standard linguistic methods. Notice also that the finding cannot be accounted for by saying that the patients have lost their knowledge of pronouns, because they must have used it for (24c). (Blumstein et al. 1983 show that lexical knowledge of this sort is indeed at the patients' disposal.)

Thus, we have here another case where data from aphasics can show how the brain cuts the syntactic pie. One last piece is missing, though: an explanation of the patients' poor performance on the "pronoun" condition. Such an account is unlikely to appear in the form of a generalization of the Trace-Deletion account of chapter 3. Yet even without it, the very fact that one approach accounts precisely for the data patterns, and the other does not, cannot be ignored.[5]

Obviously, the next step is to test further constructions, beginning with bound pronouns like the ones in (26).

(26) a. Every duck touched her neighbor.
    b. The duck touched her neighbor.
    c. Every duck touched herself.
    d. Max touched his dog, and Bill did too.
    e. Only Steve touched his friend.

The constructions tested so far show that knowledge of rule (20) and the coindexing procedure is used to exclude ungrammatical interpretations. The sentences in (26), if tested correctly, will indicate whether this knowledge is used to force bound variable readings—that is, whether or not the patients can bind a variable consistently.

Reinhart's account predicts that since the bound variable reading is always available to the patients, they should perform well above chance in a task involving the comprehension of all these constructions, despite the fact that they fail to comprehend pragmatically determined pronominal coreference. Most saliently, although failing with sentences like *The duck touched her*, they would succeed with (26b), because a bound variable reading is available there. By contrast, the standard GB approach would predict that only on sentences that involve reflexives—here, (26c)—would agrammatic aphasics achieve high levels of accuracy. Experiments designed to test these predictions are currently in preparation. Despite the difficulty of conducting these experiments—the number of controls that must be administered is rather large—they must be carried out in order to strengthen the evidential basis for the argument. Yet even at this preliminary stage the available data tend in the right direction. This is rather suggestive. At the very least, the existence of such cases indicates strongly, in my view, that evidence of the type discussed is of great value, for it may yield fruitful, and sometimes surprising, results.

4.4 Conclusion

Before concluding this chapter, I should emphasize a methodological point regarding the status of the claims made here compared to other experimentally motivated claims that are supposed to bear on linguistic models. Most of the claims based on so-called psychological evidence have been founded on reaction-time data. This kind of evidence suffers from well-known methodological problems, some of which I have already mentioned, concerning the assumptions one makes about the observed time-course of parsing and about its relation both to the grammar and to machine-time as assumed by the model. Let us look for a moment at the details of these assumptions and at the problems they raise.

These problems arise when one puts a theory of grammar to an empirical test by measuring the time-course of sentence processing. It is usually argued (see Crain and Fodor 1985; Freedman and Forster 1985) that differences in reaction-time data among constructions imply differences in the number of operations involved in the grammatical derivation of these constructions. Thus, various findings are taken to confirm some theories and falsify others. However, this may be true only if two auxiliary assumptions are made, as Berwick and Weinberg (1984) have argued quite convincingly. First, one must assume a theory of perceptual complexity that mimics, more or less, the theory of grammar. No independent motivation is usually given for this assumption. Second, one must assume a given time-value for each of the hypothesized processes, and, given that it is difficult to tease these processes apart, the value assigned to each of them remains, in many instances, a wild card. Given these points, two degrees of freedom remain unaccounted for in the time-course argument, which makes it much less compelling than one would like it to be. Indeed, as Berwick and

Weinberg show, small changes in the time-cost of a putative process may force a radically different interpretation. By contrast, the method used here makes no such assumptions. All one has to assume here is that breakdown patterns are telling a relevant story—to my mind, a plausible assumption in the framework of a realistic theory of grammar.

In conclusion, I have argued in favor of imposing a novel kind of constraint on the theory of syntax, the breakdown-compatibility constraint, which requires that it be possible to state language breakdown patterns naturally in the theory. The cases I have discussed are not necessarily the only ones, nor should they be the most important. Yet the significance of such claims is clear: if true, they impose severe restrictions on the class of biologically feasible grammars. They should thus be used for the evaluation of theoretical proposals.

Chapter 5

Neuropsychological Clues concerning the Modularity of Language

5.1 Approaches to Perception

Perceiving the world around us is a nontrivial task, in which heavy machinery is clearly needed for performance as successful as ours. This of course complicates life for students of perception. The problems they have to solve are complex, and the characterization of the perceptual machine is therefore extremely difficult. Indeed, the nature of perception has been a topic of debate for centuries, and a major breakthrough unfortunately does not seem imminent. Yet there are occasional innovations in this area—new variants of old approaches, new discoveries of what people can and cannot do, new terminology. In fact, the field has lately witnessed interesting developments, some of which are the topic of this chapter. I refer specifically to a new framework for the study of perception, Jerry Fodor's modularity thesis (1983). In section 5.2 I will present the central tenets of this approach, by way of contrasting it with one of its main opponents, known as "new look" psychology, as represented by Bruner (1973). Then I will discuss how empirical evidence gathered from the study of acquired language deficits— aphasic syndromes—can be brought to bear on the theoretical claims. I will look at the description of agrammatism, as formulated in chapter 3, and use it to motivate a neurological argument concerning the modularity of the language processor. It will turn out that there is neuropsychological evidence supporting the contention that at least the linguistic portion of our perceptual system is modular in Fodor's sense.

After World War II a new approach to perception was gradually developed in the United States. It was later known as "new look" psychology, with Jerome Bruner as its main proponent.[1] "New look" psychology was a reaction to behaviorism. And, as behaviorist psychology gained notoriety for plainly denying that mental life exists at all, "new look" psychology boldly revived mental processes as theoretical constructs; perhaps too strongly, as some would say. For, if the behaviorists refused to posit any inner processes as theoretical constructs, the "new lookers" were happy to assume many such processes, allowing for a rich and powerful cognitive theory. According to "new look" psychology, the most important properties of the perceptual system are that it is categorial, inferential, and veridical. Categorial—since all perception is actually categorization. If I show you an apple and ask you what it is, in order to say "apple" you will have to say to yourself, "Ah, this is a red-green rounded shiny object, not too hard, with a stem on top. It must be an apple." Inferential—for we have just seen how the act of categorization must be augmented with an inference: since the object has properties XYZ, and you have some background knowledge of what these properties mean, then the object must be an apple. Veridical (in a special sense)—for you can tell me what the next apple up the branch should look like.

Perception, then, is a process that involves inferences over content, background knowledge, and much more. In fact, Bruner has claimed that the determinants of perceptual readiness even include attentional factors and all the knowledge we can recruit. According to him, this is the reason for our great success in "going beyond the information given," a phrase he coined. We see a black dot on the horizon along with some specks of smoke, and we immediately recognize it as a ship. Our knowledge comes to the aid of our sensorium in a direct, unrestricted fashion. And our theory may take virtually anything as a determinant of perceptual readiness.

Against this theoretical framework, represented today by interactionists like Tyler and Marslen-Wilson in psycholinguistics and Anderson, Schank, and Simon in artificial intelligence, and by connectionists like McClelland, Hinton, and Rumelhart,[2] there emerges the modular approach. If the interactionist would allow background knowledge, mental state, mood, and so on, to penetrate our perceptual system at any given point, the modular approach would maintain just the opposite. Basically, it says this: Perception is *not* inferential (at least not in the "new look" sense); the flow of information between perceptual and inferential processes is severely restricted; attention has nothing to do with perception. In short, modularity declares its irreconcilable differences from "new look" psychology and interactionism. It then sets a program, "divide-and-conquer" style, to characterize the nature of the perceptual system, claiming that the system consists of (roughly) six "modules," one for each sense and one for language. Let me elaborate.

5.2 Modularity: Basic Properties

The central claims of the modular approach are these: Our perceptual system is modular. Each module is cognitively impenetrable, informationally encapsulated, and domain-specific, and the operation of each one is mandatory. In short, a module is a cluster concept consisting of several terms, each of which has a relatively clear explication.

Fodor maintains that our cognitive system is divided into central and peripheral portions. The former is capable of making inferences and is sensitive to attentional factors, moods, and so forth, whereas the latter—composed of the lower-level, specialized perceptual processors—is the target of the modularity thesis. Fodor thus revives the old distinction between perception and cognition that the "new look" agenda blurs. Specifically, modules—each a peripheral processor dedicated to a single domain, whether vision, hearing, or language—are impenetrable to influence from higher cognitive systems. That is, higher processes, background knowledge, mood, and so on, can apply only to the *output* of the lower processors and can never affect their operation. The classic, most powerful examples come from the visual domain. These are illusions (or paradoxes) such as the Muller-Lyer illusion shown in (1).

(1)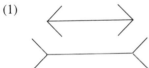

The lower line, with the extended edges, looks longer than the upper one, and even if you measure them and become convinced that they are actually the same length, you will still perceive them as unequal. You simply can't help perceiving them the way you do: background knowledge cannot penetrate perceptual processes, and you are forever captive to your visual analyzer, which, as it happens, is cheated by circumstances. This is, then, the content of the cognitive impenetrability claim.

The second major claim of modularity concerns the informational encapsulation of each module. According to this claim, if a lower process has knowledge in its possession, then higher processes have no access to this knowledge, which is encapsulated within the module in question. For example, if you believe that we possess linguistic knowledge in the form of grammatical rules and that this knowledge is instrumental in the on-line analysis of incoming sentences, then the modularity thesis would claim that we can use this knowledge but cannot report to others, or to ourselves, anything about its nature. That is to say, when asked about the grammatical status of a sentence, we can always reply quite reliably,

"This string is grammatical; that one is ungrammatical," but when asked about the rules invoked in the process by which we decided, we are unable to list them. Grammatical knowledge is thus part and parcel of the language module, and therefore, we cannot have conscious access to it.

The third major claim of modularity concerns the mandatory nature of modular processing. Once a modular process is initiated, it must run its entire course. There is no way to stop it in the midst of processing. Just think of your knee-jerk reflex: you can't help extending your leg upon being hit below your kneecap, nor can you stop your leg partway through the extension. Perceptual analysis, Fodor claims, is just as reflexive. (For an experimental investigation of this claim in the phonetic domain, see Miller 1986.)

A lower perceptual unit, then, has these properties (and some other, less important ones). Since the modularity thesis is an empirical claim, it should be tested; and since it is a very general claim, it must be tested in many cognitive domains.

5.3   The Structure of the Argument

What does it take to demonstrate the modularity of an input system? For each putative property of a modular system the argument is different. The most interesting are naturally the properties concerning restrictions on the flow of information. I will therefore concentrate on cognitive impenetrability and informational encapsulation. In each instance I will demonstrate modularity by providing an empirical argument that the cognitive system is irrational in a particular way.

An input system is said to be cognitively impenetrable if higher cognitive processes can never interfere with its operation. Therefore, a case must be found where such interference would be beneficial to the organism, because it would improve performance on some task. Now, if we find that no such interference occurs in spite of these considerations, then we are forced to assume that there is an architectural barrier that blocks the higher cognitive process from influencing the lower input system. The latter is thus cognitively impenetrable.

To demonstrate the informational encapsulation property, we want to show the reverse: that a higher process cannot utilize information that is stored in a lower system. Technically, the argument has the following form: (1) Construct a task, and present a task analysis according to which a specific pattern of performance will be observed that indicates that if the subject has certain information available, there is an (optimal) algorithm that restricts the solution space, speeds up processing, or reduces error, depending on the nature of the task. (2) Show that the subject does not behave as expected and that one of two interpretations is forced: either the subject is behaving irrationally, or the subject deviates from the algorithm constructed by the task analysis. (3) Show that the locus of the deviation is the link between the information and the operations necessary to carry out the task.

In other words, to demonstrate modularity in informational flow, it is necessary to demonstrate irrationality, which is explicable only in terms of an informational gap.[3]

Take a well-known finding that is taken to support the modularity of lexical access, as proposed first by Forster (1979): Swinney's (1979) experiment. This experiment uses the Cross-Modal-Lexical-Decision paradigm, which is based on auditory presentation of sentences, and then a lexical decision task to a string of letters presented on a screen. The visually presented string is given in the midst of the sentence, that is, at a designated point during the presentation of the auditory stimulus. Swinney shows that left context (what the subject hears before the target word) does not facilitate lexical access to words that are "predictable" from it, when compared to other words. This conclusion is based on investigating the time the subject takes to make a lexical decision on pairs of words, as follows: The subject hears a string like *The FBI agent searched the room for BUGS...*, where either *SPY* or *ANT* is presented visually for lexical decision. If left context helps in lexical access, then SPY should be primed (everything else being equal). Yet this does not happen, which suggests that lexical access is never influenced by background knowledge, no matter how recent it is.

In other words, either the system deliberately ignores available information—thus exhibiting irrational behavior—or, more likely, the flow of information is restricted: lower processes (lexical access in Swinney's case) cannot be penetrated by higher ones, and higher processes have no access to information stored in lower parts of the system. Swinney demonstrates part of what is needed to prove that informational encapsulation holds: he shows that lexical access cannot use background knowledge provided in left context.

I think I have a good instance of the above general argument for the language domain. That is, if my data are reliable and my argument valid, then the processor dedicated to the on-line analysis of incoming sentences—the syntactic parser—constitutes a module in Fodor's sense. The evidence I will present comes from examining the syntactic abilities of agrammatic patients.

5.4   An Argument from Aphasia

The argument has the following form. Recall the claim from chapter 3 that the linguistic performance of agrammatic patients on comprehension tasks demonstrates a selective impairment of some syntactic functions and that as a result, their comprehension is based on both syntactic processing and heuristics that are invoked to compensate for the loss. The account is thus based on an interaction between syntactic (linguistic) and general cognitive (nonlinguistic) knowledge. Here I will look at the details of this interaction and show that it is severely restricted: heuristic processes can apply only *after* the syntactic processor had completed its job (which, in the case of these patients, it cannot do adequately). This result will bear on the claim that a module, and the linguistic module in particular, is cognitively impenetrable, that is, that higher processes can never interfere with the action of lower-level perceptual mechanisms—nonlinguistic processes must wait (if my account is correct) for the completion of grammar-based analysis. I will further show that my account of agrammatic comprehension bears on the claim of informational encapsulation, namely, that the content of lower processors is inaccessible to higher, central systems. I will do so by demonstrating that if the cognitive system had access to grammatical knowledge, and not just to the representations that the parser outputs, it would behave differently, and agrammatic patients would perform better than they actually do. In other words, the patients' performance is either based on irrational considerations or supported by a modularly organized system. These two results will thus constitute empirical evidence from neuropsychology in support of the modularity thesis. (For a different view of modularity, and evidence bearing on it, see Poizner, Bellugi, and Klima 1986.)

The formal description of comprehension in agrammatic aphasia assumes an interaction between incomplete grammatical representations and a nongrammatical heuristic. This heuristic is invoked in order to "salvage" NPs that cannot receive thematic assignment normally. It is necessary because patients are faced with a task that forces them to map every NP in a given sentence onto a representation of a depiction of a real-world event. As a result, they are forced to assign a semantic role to each NP. When they fail to derive the semantic role from the grammatically assigned theta-role, they assign one by the default heuristic.

Most important here is that the domain of application of the heuristic is highly restricted: it applies only to those NPs that are not assigned a theta-role by the grammar, that is, to NPs in nonthematic positions. In other words, a condition defined in purely syntactic terms determines whether or not the Default Principle is activated. Moreover, this condition cannot be met unless an analysis of a whole clause is available, because the definition of the heuristic's domain of application involves the term "nonthematic position," which cannot be determined otherwise. Hence, the strategy cannot apply anywhere but *after* the parser has completed recovering whatever structural description it is capable of recovering from the input string. If the condition for its application is met, the heuristic assigns agenthood to the NP in question. It is important to note that the heuristic definitely comes from nonlinguistic knowledge sources. As shown in chapter 3, the attempt to state it in a fashion that is sensitive to linguistic knowledge (that is, to the theta-grid of the verb in question) fails on descriptive grounds, forcing the alternative conclusion that it is a general cognitive strategy that assigns semantic roles to position regardless of the thematic properties of the predicate.

What are the implications of this arrangement for the structure of the language processor and in particular for the relation between syntactic processes and nonsyntactic knowledge? The question is, of course, whether or not the former are susceptible to influence from the latter. This is important, because an answer to this question can determine a crucial property of the modularity issue: the "cognitive impenetrability" of processes dedicated to the formal analysis of input strings. Given that heuristic strategies of the type we have been discussing arise from surface regularities of strings and from semantic and other knowledge, and not from linguistic knowledge, if these strategies were permitted to interfere with the work of the parser, rather than apply to its output only, then we would conclude that the parser is not "cognitively impenetrable"; hence, it would be nonmodular by Fodor's criteria. This is the position that Bever (1970) effectively maintains in his formulation of strategies. For him they can apply at any point— in fact, they can apply competitively with the grammar. But the description of agrammatism proposed in chapter 3 suggests the opposite, namely, that the language recognition device is impenetrable and that heuristics stemming from nonlinguistic sources may have access only to its output and cannot interfere with its operation. This follows from the claim that the heuristic strategy applies only to phrases that have particular properties (that is, to NPs that are in nonthematic positions). As such, it can *only* apply to the output of the parser. Thus, the deficient parser must first compute whatever it can of the representation of the clause, and only afterward can the strategy apply.

In fact, if this account is correct, then the application of the strategy sometimes results in the violation of grammatical principles. However, independent experimental evidence indicates that agrammatic aphasics know the principles, as demonstrated by their ability to detect violations of them in a grammaticality judgment task. (See Linebarger, Schwartz, and Saffran 1983, especially the condition called "gapless relatives"; also see Sproat 1986.) It follows that the patients in a sense invoke the heuristic strategy in spite of the grammatical knowledge they possess.

A notable example involves the Theta Criterion, which ensures congruence between properties of assigners and assignees. Clearly, if the theta-role agent is assigned to two NPs, this violates the dictum of the Theta Criterion that each role may be assigned only once. It follows that the strategy does not necessarily observe these principles, even though they are available at the time the phrase marker is constructed, that is, during the parse. This means that nonlinguistic strategies have access only to *representations* that the parser outputs and not to the grammatical *principles* (or rules) that the parser observes. The strategies are thus barred from using the grammar for guidance.

If this is true, then we have a very strong argument for the existence of the second central property of modular systems in the language processor: informational encapsulation. If the strategy had access to grammatical principles, it might not violate them, and aphasic patients would, in some cases, be better off. Consider, for example, the passive case in (2).

(2) Normal
    assignment   theme   agent

                    $[_{NP_1}$ the boy] was pushed by $[_{NP_2}$ the girl]
    Agrammatic   agent   agent
    assignment

According to the account in chapter 3, patients make the assignment to NP_1 heuristically, and to NP_2 grammatically. The heuristic thus applies without self-monitoring, so to speak. Yet, had they acted in their own best interest, the patients would have withheld application of the strategy in this case and would have attempted to augment their incomplete representation differently. They would have used the grammar to assign the role of agent to the object of the preposition *by*, and since they are unable to assign a theta-role to the subject because the trace is deleted, they could have inferred, using their grammar, that the subject must be theme. Were this the case, then their performance on passives would be indistinguishable from normal performance. They would succeed in compensating for their loss by making an inference, thus assigning the theta-role to the "dangling" NP in subject position indirectly. But they do not seem to be doing that. Rather, they seem to invoke a strategy that assigns the agent role to the subject of the passive, and the result is chance performance. Using the strategy is therefore not always the rational thing for patients to do, yet they seem to use it, sometimes, in a self-defeating fashion. What is the reason for this irrational behavior? We have a natural explanation for this if we assume that the syntactic parser is informationally encapsulated: nothing can interfere with its action, and the information to which it has access is not available to processes external to it. On this view, the grammatical principles that are violated are simply inaccessible to the strategy.

Here is another way of saying the same thing, in a more detailed fashion. In the case of passive, if the flow of information were unrestricted, then patients would have the information shown in (3) available, as premises.

(3)   P1: The verb has two theta-roles: agent, theme.
       P2: The string to be analyzed has two NPs.
       P3: NP_2 = agent

If they had access to all this information, they would be able to make the deduction shown in (4).

(4) NP_1 = theme

For optimal performance, application of the inference should suppress the use of the strategy, because such use would lead to aberrant performance. However, patients do not suppress the strategy, instead assigning the agent role to NP_1. This amounts to irrational behavior on their part. The first thing we must establish is the reason for this behavior. Assuming our patients to be rational, we are left with two possibilities: either their deductive abilities are lost, or one (or more) of the premises are inaccessible to them at the right time. Our general knowledge of agrammatic aphasics indicates, I believe, that their deductive abilities are preserved. Had these abilities been impaired, the patients' daily functioning would be hindered. This, however, seems not to be the case. It follows, then, that the problem lies with the premises in (3). But which one is missing at the point where the strategy applies?

Following our account of agrammatism, P3 must be available, because the patients assign an agent theta-role to NP_2. Similarly, P2 must be available: the patients know that the strings contain two NPs. It follows that P1 is unavailable—in other words, that knowledge of the thematic properties of predicators is missing. But here a potential contradiction arises. We have assumed that most of the thematic representation patients have is constructed by their use of thematic knowledge, yet now we are saying that thematic knowledge is unavailable. The way out of this paradox is to assume that although the thematic properties of predicators are available to the parser at the time it constructs a syntactic analysis for the sentence, this knowledge is unavailable to processes that are outside the parser. In other words, the strategy has access to the output of the parser (in our case a thematically incomplete representation), but it cannot look at the grammatical knowledge (principles, rules, and so forth) that the parser uses. This conclusion is further supported by the observation that the Theta Criterion is violated in agrammatic comprehension, even though in judging the grammaticality of sentences, patients show that they actually possess this grammatical principle. It follows that the strategy lies outside the jurisdiction of the Theta Criterion and therefore cannot use it.

The same form of reasoning just applied to the passive holds for all the constructions on which the formal characterization of agrammatism has been based. We are therefore forced to conclude that grammatical principles that the agrammatic aphasic's parser possesses are unavailable to higher cognitive processes. This is what makes some of these processes "dumb." The informational encapsulation property is thus satisfied.

Note that this is the reverse of Swinney's argument. Swinney shows that a certain kind of information (in his case, contextual) is initially not available but later (some 300 milliseconds downstream) becomes available. This is a case, then, of initial unconstrained, "automatic" access and later constrained, directed access. By contrast, what is initially observed in the case we have been looking at is an activity that is motivated by grammatical considerations, that is, the construction of an incomplete phrase marker, as guided by the grammar; the later activity of augmentative processes (that is, the heuristic strategy) is not guided by grammatical knowledge, and in fact these processes do not have access to such knowledge.

In sum, then, the heuristic strategy comes into play only after the parser has completed its work, because the strategy's domain of application is defined syntactically and without a full syntactic analysis a phrase complying with this definition cannot be identified. This satisfies the requirement of cognitive impenetrability. On the other hand, the application of the strategy is completely blind to lower-level grammatical knowledge; if the strategy had access to this knowledge, its operation would improve the patients' performance. This satisfies the requirement of informational encapsulation.

At this stage it might be argued that since aphasic deficits represent a partial failure of the language system, arguments like the one just adduced cannot hold: this failure may have caused unknown changes in the system, with the result that nothing can be learned about it from the data we have examined. This argument is misguided, however. Since by assumption the deficit lies in the linguistic system, one would expect a deficient processor to use any piece of data to which it can have access. In particular, if it had access to semantic information, we would surely expect it to use that information. If the account I have presented is correct, however, then even in cases like agrammatic aphasia, where the language system is partially disrupted, the parser is barred from using nonsyntactic information. It therefore seems that the fact that the evidence is neuropsychological does not weaken the argument but rather strengthens it. It demonstrates how research into language pathologies can provide precious evidence that could not be obtained otherwise.

Thus, the available evidence suggests that the human parsing device has two central properties of the type of modular system that Fodor proposes: any knowledge external to it (in particular, nonlinguistic knowledge) does not enter into its considerations, and knowledge it possesses cannot be used by systems external to it. This seems to be so even in extreme conditions such as cases of language impairment. And if these claims are correct for the impaired comprehension device of agrammatic aphasics, then they are certainly true for the normal, fully functioning, human comprehension device.

Chapter 6

Language Acquisition and Language Breakdown: A Reappraisal

6.1 Introduction

Any normal adult is taken to be the average owner of a language faculty. It is the linguistic knowledge of this organism that theories of language structure are about. Apart from individual differences, from which these theories tend to abstract away, there are two notable deviations from the average speaker. The first is the developing child, who has not yet had the time to reach full-fledged linguistic ability, and the second is the aphasic, who was a good representative of the community of speakers prior to the illness that caused the aphasia but has become linguistically incapacitated to some degree.

The relation between these states in which the human linguistic abilities are incomplete has intrigued thinkers for many years. In the literature of the past century one idea recurs in a number of versions: developing children learn language in the inverse order that aphasics "unlearn" it. Put differently, if there are stages in the acquisition of language, then there should be a corresponding aphasic state (or perhaps syndrome) for each. This idea was first expressed in Ribot's Law (Ribot 1883), according to which the later a piece of knowledge is acquired, the more susceptible it is to be lost in language disorder. In our century this type of thesis has been associated with Jakobson's (1941) influential Regression Hypothesis, a much-discussed claim in the past decade or so (see Caramazza and Zurif 1978a; Hyams 1986b). In this chapter I will reexamine this type of claim in light of the view of language deficits developed in previous chapters, as well as certain current views on language learning. Through a detailed discussion of properties of developing and deficient language faculties I will attempt to assess the coherence of such claims, their empirical adequacy, and their relevance to theoretical issues.

The chapter is organized as follows. First I discuss in general the similarities and differences between development and dissolution of language. Next I examine the relationship between the two cases with respect to two theoretical proposals: the Regression Hypothesis and the more recent Subset Principle (Baker 1979; Dell 1981; Berwick 1982; Manzini and Wexler 1987). Finally I take up a particular theoretical issue regarding language development.

6.2 Acquisition and Dissolution: Similarities and Differences

The nativist approach to the language faculty provides many dimensions along which to compare linguistic systems that deviate from the normal in the two senses considered here. In this section I take issues that have been discussed in detail with respect to one area and extend the discussion to the other. This approach both provides a set of properties for the comparison between language acquisition and language breakdown and points to the fact that some important questions concerning language deficits are still unanswered.

The first question concerns the relation between the grammars of the impoverished states and Universal Grammar (UG). That is, do the grammars of the developing child and the aphasic constitute possible human grammars? For developing children, it seems, the answer is yes. Pinker (1984), for instance, argues quite convincingly that the null hypothesis must be that the child's grammar is as close to the adult's as possible. Hyams (1986a) points out that since the developing child is equipped with principles of UG that are taken to be innate, it follows that each intermediate grammar that the child possesses must be constrained by these principles.[1] And since the characterization of a possible human grammar is exactly the requirement that it be so constrained, then all child grammars are possible—albeit otherwise unattested—human languages. Therefore, if the development of language consists in the successive possession of a series of grammars $G_1 ... G_i ... G_n$, the first referring to the initial state (prior to any exposure to the linguistic environment) and the last referring to the steady state (the adult grammar), then any G_i, $1 \leq i \leq n$ is a possible grammar in that it abides by the constraints specified by UG.

Although the answer is rather straightforward in the case of children, it is not in the case of aphasics. The considerations in this instance are substantially more complex and depend on the nature of the aphasic impairment. As mentioned in chapter 3, the impairment in agrammatism may be due to a loss of grammatical principles (from either the core or the periphery), or disruption of the processors that implement the grammar, or both. In each case, however, violation of (at least some) principles of UG is permitted. If such a principle is lost through brain damage, then it may certainly be violated: all the strings it rules out exclusively are now in the language. However, if the grammar is left intact and a processor is disrupted, one can imagine cases where grammatical principles are violated because the process responsible for implementing or observing them is not available. Yet in this case it would be misleading to say that the principle itself is violated (see Sproat 1986 and Grodzinsky 1986b for an exchange on this issue). To say now that the aphasic's grammar is different from those permitted by UG would contradict the initial assumption. One can only say that the sentences accepted by this implementation violate universal principles—a weaker claim. In sum, only if a grammatical principle is demonstrably lost can we say that the aphasic possesses a language that is not a possible human language. And, since our discussion of the source of the impairment in agrammatism was inconclusive, we are not in a position to take a stand on this issue. We are certainly not in a position to make statements with respect to other syndromes. The little available evidence on agrammatism seems to suggest, though, that the impairment is not to the underlying grammar. If this is the case, then the agrammatic possesses an underlying grammar that is permitted by UG.

If we adopt a version of the Regression Hypothesis, however, another possibility opens up—namely, that aphasia is a mirror image of development. If so, and if language learning is nothing but parameter fixing, then aphasia is a loss of parametric values; hence, aphasic grammars clearly conform to principles of UG. This possibility is discussed in detail below.

Next we should look at the developing and deficient grammars from the point of view of the learning paradigm that is commonly assumed in generative grammar. According to this framework, learning is a function that maps from (exclusively positive) linguistic input onto a grammar. That is, children are taken to be extremely sensitive to positive data and to move from one stage to the next (from G_i to G_{i+1}; see Pinker 1984; Hyams 1986a) on the basis of the strings they are presented with; yet they are totally insensitive to negative data or correction, at least in the syntactic domain (Brown and Hanlon 1970). Predictably, the situation is less clear in aphasia, yet certain questions can already be answered quite decisively. Suppose, to take the most extreme case, that aphasics lose a part of their language faculty, consisting of both language-particular rules and universal constraints. Are they then open to positive evidence? That is, can they reacquire the missing pieces just through casual exposure? This seems most unlikely for two reasons. First, the functional loss is due to *physical* loss of neural tissue, supposedly making aphasics worse off in some way than children. Second, the language faculty is fixed around puberty; beyond that stage humans can no longer acquire a language as a mother tongue (Lenneberg 1967; Fromkin et al. 1974). It would be most surprising if, under these conditions, aphasics were to learn from positive evidence; and it would follow that if any relearning is observed, it does not occur through the language faculty itself but instead is mediated by nonlinguistic cognitive resources. These two issues are clearly related to remediation of the aphasias. Unless sensitivity to either positive or, more likely, negative evidence is demonstrated, one cannot conclude that a particular therapeutic method is efficacious.[2] I am aware of no such demonstrably effective method of treatment.

A final comparative issue concerns the size of the language the child or aphasic possess. We will look at this issue in detail in section 6.3.4. For now, suffice it to say that when issues of size are relevant—that is, when a grammatical principle is in the domain of the Subset Principle—then the language generated by the child's grammar is, by this principle, a subset of the adult language, whereas the aphasic's constitutes a superset, if the aphasic is deficient in a sense relevant to this particular domain.

These observations can be conveniently summarized in table 6.1.

Table 6.1

	Acquisition	Aphasia
Relation to the final state G_n	pre–	post–
Sensitivity to positive data	+	–
Sensitivity to negative data	–	+
Possession of a humanly possible grammar	+	?
Language size	$\leq L(G_n)$	$\geq L(G_n)$
Flexibility of the language faculty	+	–

6.3 Learnability and Dissolution of Language

6.3.1 The Regression Hypothesis

The fact that both children and aphasics are "deviant" linguistically has led many to believe that a deep analogy must hold between their language systems. Roman Jakobson (1941) made a simple yet bold claim. After defining a set of phonological distinctive features, which he claimed constituted a universal inventory, he identified a hierarchy among them. He then related this hierarchy, in opposite orders, to acquisition and dissolution. Thus, if the ability to distinguish between [+labial] and [–labial] appears in the child prior to the ability to distinguish between [+voiced] and [–voiced], then Jakobson's account contends that the latter is higher on the hierarchy than the former, hence dependent on it. Consequently, in aphasia (the account continues) loss of the ability to identify "labiality" as a feature necessarily entails loss of the ability to identify "voice" or "voicelessness." This claim is known as the Regression Hypothesis, according to which the order of dissolution of the linguistic system is identical to, yet opposite in direction from, the order of acquisition. Formally, as shown in (1), it means that for every grammar G_i, $1 \leq i \leq n$, that the developing child adopts and rejects (except G_n, the grammar of the steady state) in the sequence $G_1,...,G_n$, there is a corresponding aphasic grammar G'_j, $1 \leq j \leq n$, such that $G'_1 = G_n$ and $G_i = G'_j$ if and only if $i = n - j$. Notice that the number and identity of the grammars in $G_1,...,G_n$ equal the number and identity of the grammars in $G'_1,...,G'_n$ and that the last requirement ensures inverse order of the sequences.

(1) Regression Hypothesis

Let $S = G_1,...,G_n$ be a sequence of all the child grammars, and $S' = G'_1,...,G'_m$ a sequence of all aphasic grammars. Then for every $1 \leq i \leq n$, $1 \leq j \leq m$:

a. $m = n$

b. $G_i = G'_j$ if and only if $i = n - j$

This formulation raises an immediate question concerning the notion "aphasic grammar": though the concept of "stages" is relatively clear with respect to acquisition, it isn't with respect to aphasia. Does it mean that an aphasic syndrome will be found to correspond to each stage of language acquisition? Does it refer to stages through which every aphasic who is at a dynamic stage of the disease must pass? Or does it perhaps refer to degrees of severity in the same syndrome? (2) lists these possible interpretations in relation to the Regression Hypothesis.

(2) The notion "aphasic grammar" will be interpreted as follows:

a. For every G'_j, $1 \leq j \leq n$, in (1) there is an *aphasic syndrome*, and for every syndrome there is a G'_j.

b. For every G'_j, $1 \leq j \leq n$, in (1) there is a *stage of recovery* in a given aphasic syndrome, and for every such stage there is a G'_j.

c. For every G'_j, $1 \leq j \leq n$, in (1) there is a *degree of severity* in a given aphasic syndrome, and for every such degree there is a G'_j.

Clearly, for each choice in (2) there is a distinct Regression Hypothesis. Indeed, all of them are represented in the literature. For instance, Wepman and Jones (1964) have claimed that, on a particular scale, the stages of acquisition parallel the variety of aphasic syndromes, thus picking the Regression Hypothesis with the definition of aphasic grammar in (2a). Goodglass (1978) argues against the empirical adequacy of this claim, pointing out, as a counterexample, that a recovering Wernicke's aphasic never passes through a stage of agrammatism. As stated, his argument is invalid, of course, since the notion of aphasic grammar he refers to is (2b) and he and Wepman and Jones are thus examining different versions of the Regression Hypothesis. Caramazza and Zurif (1978b) adopt the definition in (2c) and state without justification that it is the only one possible, writing that

at most,...the regression hypothesis would appear to apply only within specific aphasic syndromes....The critical aphasic variable in the development-dissolution equation is the severity of impairment within each syndrome, and any parallels between language acquisition and language breakdown will hold only between stages of development of specific language components and severity of disruption of like components. (p. 146)

These authors adduce evidence that in their view falsifies the Regression Hypothesis.

Several points should be noted here. First, the Regression Hypothesis makes sense only when referring to sequences of grammars (or performance patterns interpretable in grammatical terms). Second, the sequence of aphasic grammars can be defined in a variety of ways, and since this issue has never been discussed in detail, there is considerable confusion about it in the literature. Third, for the Regression Hypothesis to stand, it must be shown that the child and the aphasic have the same number of grammars and that each child grammar has a corresponding aphasic grammar. It is not surprising that no proponent of the hypothesis has done this. For one thing, none of them has assumed a coherent theory of language learning to determine the nature of the sequence S, against which the findings from aphasia, presumably characterizing the sequence S', can be seriously evaluated.

In the formulation in (1), stages of both language acquisition and language loss are characterized by the grammars of the observable language, even though the literature might occasionally contain a slightly different characterization. In fact, Ribot's Law, the original formulation, states that the later a *form* is acquired, the more susceptible it is to impairment.

Jakobson (1941) fashioned his claim similarly. For him, each stage is represented by a particular phonological distinctive feature, and the aphasic loses the ability to distinguish between distinctive features. Thus, the two strings in (3) will be equivalent for the aphasic.

(3)   a. reflector
      b. lefrectol

This means that there is at least one string that is ungrammatical for the normal speaker but perfectly acceptable for the aphasic. According to Jakobson, the sequence in (3b) would sound well-formed to the aphasic. He would therefore claim that if there is a child who is as yet unable to distinguish between (3a) and (3b), then there is a corresponding aphasic. Yet this kind of claim is equivalent to the statement in (1), because the acquisition of a distinction (or a rule) reflects a move from one grammatical stage G_i to its successor G_{i+1}.

Similarly, Hyams's (1986b) proposal that the Regression Hypothesis is true for inflectional *forms* is translatable to a version of (1). Specifically, Hyams seeks to reconcile apparently conflicting observations in the acquisition literature concerning the cross-linguistic description of the development of inflection. In some languages, like English, inflections are initially missing from the child's speech. In others, like Italian and Hebrew, they are not. Hyams proposes a parametric account of these phenomena, according to which the lexical well-formedness of a stem would determine its rate of acquisition and patterns of omission. She then observes that a similar claim has been made for agrammatism (Grodzinsky 1984a, reformulated in chapter 3) and proposes that the value of this parameter is fixed early cross-linguistically but that rules of agreement are acquired late. In her view, this proposal not only explains the cross-linguistic data she presents but also confirms Jakobson's claims, because the same elements are highly susceptible to disruption.[3]

In view of this wide disagreement, it may be useful to reexamine the Regression Hypothesis. In fact, without a precise statement of both the Regression Hypothesis and a theory of learning no serious evaluation can be undertaken. In order to arrive at such a statement, we must first take a look at language learning.

6.3.2   Conceptual Issues in Language Learning

The basic problems here follow from the assumption, widely accepted among students of language acquisition today, that in learning a language, children have no access to "negative evidence." That is, children are insensitive to correction and thus can never be told that a given string is ungrammatical (see Brown and Hanlon 1970; later works also substantiate this position). It follows, then, that children learn languages by being confronted with "positive evidence"— grammatical sentences only. Now, given that there is a fair amount of idiosyncrasy in any given language, how can children ever learn certain lexical exceptions without being sensitive to correction at all?

This question was first raised in linguistics by Baker (1979). He presented the contrasts shown in (4) and (5).

(4)   a. John gave a book to Mary.

   b. John gave Mary a book.

(5) a. John donated a book to Mary.
    b. *John donated Mary a book.

The similarity of meaning between (4a) and (4b), Baker observed, suggests that they are related by a rule, possibly a transformational one. Now, suppose that this rule exists. Then, since *give* and *donate* have similar meanings, as well as a dative object, how can the child ever know, without having access to negative evidence, that the latter cannot have a double object? That is, upon being exposed to both forms of *give*, what would prevent the child from assuming that *donate* belongs to the same class of verbs, thus forming double object constructions with *donate* as well?

Children's (immature) grammar cannot be such that their language contains ungrammatical strings (that is, strings that are inadmissible in the adult language). If their grammar did contain ungrammatical strings, how could they ever retreat to the adult boundary, without ever being corrected? Baker considered various solutions to this problem. For example, he proposed that the relation between (4a) and (4b) is arbitrary and that there is no need to state a rule and then block its application in certain instances.

The important problem in the present context is the problem of retreat. If our theory of language is stated in terms of general rules with lexical exceptions, then the child has a language that is not a subset of the adult language (that is, it contains at least one ungrammatical string). However, under the assumption that negative evidence plays no role in language acquisition, this theory becomes unlearnable and thus fails to satisfy a basic requirement that any realistic theory must meet. From the point of view of learnability, then, linguistic theory is at a crossroads here. Either it has a rule with exceptions, in which case the question is how the child ever learns the exception, being exposed to positive data only, or it has no rule, in which case a significant generalization—about the dative alternation—is missed.

Now consider a possible solution first proposed by Dell (1981) and later developed by Berwick (1982). Dell observed that just like syntax, phonology exhibits generalizations that cannot be stated without assuming exceptions. French, for example, has a rule by which a word-final liquid is optionally dropped before a pause or a consonant, if preceded by an obstruent. This is exemplified in (6):

(6) *Word*   *Pronunciation*
    a. quelle table   [keltabl] or [keltab]
    b. quel arbre   [kelarbr] or [kelarb]

As (7) shows, however, there are exceptions to this generalization.

(7) qui parle   [kiparl] but not *[kipar]

The question is how to maintain the generalization without constructing an unlearnable grammar (or alternatively, a grammar that can be learned only if access to "positive" data is assumed). Dell proposed a solution according to which the learner, upon being confronted with data, adopts a learning strategy that assumes the grammar that generates the smallest language. He proposed it as a principle governing acquisition and formulated it as shown in (8).

(8) Whenever there are two competing grammars generating languages of which one is a proper subset of the other, the learning strategy of the child is to select the less inclusive one. (Dell 1981, 34)

Dell then showed how the two possible rules governing the liquid-deletion cases (the "two competing grammars" of (8)) generate sets of strings that are in an inclusion relation, in that one of them excludes more strings than the other, even though some of the excluded strings are actually grammatical. These, Dell said, will be admitted into the grammar once presented to the child. The consequence of Dell's claims is that the learning strategy that children must assume in order to acquire the rules of their language without negative evidence is that of going from the grammar that generates the smallest set of strings, up to the adult grammar that generates a larger set. Moving on to a larger set will occur after being confronted with new evidence, suggesting a principled revision of the grammar currently possessed. Berwick (1982) has named this strategy the *Subset Principle*. According to this principle, at each stage of immaturity, developing children have a grammar generating a language that is always subset of the adult grammar. Let us now look at one particular case where this principle can be applied, taken from Manzini and Wexler 1987.

6.3.3   The Subset Principle

6.3.3.1   The Formal Statement and Its Scope   Looking at the issue from a slightly different viewpoint, Manzini and Wexler (1987) offer a full-fledged formulation of the Subset Principle. They observe that in a parameter-setting framework such as the one followed here, different values of parameters may result in languages that vary in size. That is, if our goal is to construct a theory that would account, among other things, for the differences between languages, and if these differences can be explained by appealing to parameters along which languages vary, then the process of learning is nothing but setting the values of the parameters according to the sentences to which the child is casually exposed. Under such a conception of learning it is appropriate to ask what the relation is between the values of a given parameter. If there were a parameter such that the languages defined by its possible values would stand in a subset relation to one another, learners would have a problem. Their task is to converge *exactly* on their language, because no negative evidence is allowed that would enable them to backtrack in case they passed its boundaries (that is, generated an ungrammatical string). Therefore, there must be a strategy that will allow children to pick exactly the right parametric value. Manzini and Wexler propose that this strategy is the Subset Principle, which they formalize as shown in (9) (their (38)).

(9) *Subset Principle*

Let p be a parameter with values $p_1,...,p_n,f_p$ a learning function, and D a set of data. Then for every p_i, $1 \le i \le n$,

$f_p(D) = p_i$ if and only if

a. $D \subseteq L(p_i)$ and

b. for every p_j, $1 \le j \le n$, if $D \subseteq L(p_j)$, then $L(p_i) \subseteq L(p_j)$.

This statement means that a learning function f_p that maps data D (input strings) onto a parameter p (by fixing its value) will pick the value p_i if and only if two conditions are met: (1) the data D are included in the language defined by the particular choice p_i; (2) if more than one value of the parameter can be chosen on the basis of the data, then the learning function will choose the value that defines the smallest possible language.

Two important points emerge so far. First, the Subset Principle is a learning strategy that may be instrumental in solving two aspects of the problem posed by the inaccessibility of negative evidence: the problem of lexical exceptions within a given language, and the problem of converging on the right parametric value so as to avoid overgeneration from which there is no retreat in the absence of negative evidence. Second, the scope of application of this principle is limited: conceivably, there are parameters that do not have the desirable property that their values define languages that are proper subsets of one another. Indeed, as Hyams (1986a) has shown, there are parameters (in her case, AG/PRO or pro-drop) that define languages whose set relation is intersection; that is, they define a common set of constructions, but each also defines constructions that are not defined by the other. Given this situation, in which some parameters have values that define languages related by inclusion and some do not, how can one distinguish between the two kinds? Manzini and Wexler answer this question by stating a condition on the application of the Subset Principle: the Subset Condition, shown in (10) (Manzini and Wexler's (43)), which defines the principle's domain.

(10) *Subset Condition*

Given the parameter p with values $p_1,...,p_n$, for every p_i and p_j, $1 \le i, j \le n$, either $L(p_i) \subseteq L(p_j)$ or $L(p_j) \subseteq L(p_i)$.

The Subset Condition thus defines a relation between two languages: for two values i, j, $1 \le i, j \le n$, the languages defined by each must be related in such a way that either the language defined by the choice of the value i is a subset of the language defined by the choice of the value j, or vice versa. Parameters such as Hyams's AG/PRO (pro-drop) are undefined here, which puts them outside the scope of the Subset Principle.

Thus, application of the Subset Principle to the domain defined by the Subset Condition is said to solve the problem of overgeneration in the absence of negative data. For the Subset Principle, applied to its domain, is a learning strategy that picks the correct value of a parameter when confronted with positive evidence. Retreat is never necessary because acquisition always progresses from the smaller to the larger language. In the next section I demonstrate how applying this principle yields empirically desirable results.

6.3.3.2   The Subset Principle and Binding Theory   As a concrete example of the Subset Principle, Manzini and Wexler work out the details of an issue in binding theory. They begin by assuming Binding Conditions A and B as stated by Chomsky (1981).

(11) A. An anaphor is bound in its governing category.

   B. A pronominal is free in its governing category.

(12) α binds β iff

   α c-commands β and α and β are coindexed.

(13) γ is a governing category for α iff

   γ is the minimal category that contains α and a governor for α and has a subject.

These conditions hold for English and for a number of core cases in other languages. However, Manzini and Wexler point out that they are sometimes violated in Italian, a language that differs from English. Thus, they hold for many Italian sentences, such as (14a–c), yet for others, such as (14d–e), they do not. ((14a–e) are Manzini and Wexler's (4)–(8).)

(14) a. Alice$_j$ sapeva che Mario$_i$ aveva guardato sè$_{i/*j}$ nello specchio.
       Alice Knew that Mario had   looked at Refl in the mirror
   b. Alice$_j$ pensava che Mario$_i$ avesse   guardato sè$_{i/*j}$ nello specchio.
       Alice thought that Mario had(subj.) looked at Refl in the mirror
   c. Alice$_j$ disse a Mario$_i$ di guardare sè$_{i/*j}$ nello specchio.
       Alice told   Mario   to look at Refl in the mirror
   d. Alice$_j$ vide Mario$_i$ guardare sè$_{i/j}$ nello specchio.
       Alice saw Mario look at Refl in the mirror

e. Alice$_j$ guardò   i ritratti di se$_{i/j}$ di Mario$_i$
Alice looked at portraits of Refl of Mario
'Alice looked at Mario's portraits of Refl.'

Since (14a–c) overlap with their English counterparts, the assumptions in (11)–(13) correctly account for them. However, they do not account for (14d–e). Manzini and Wexler notice that the contrast can be accounted for in terms of a different definition of "governing category." Specifically, in (14d–e) there is no need for a subject in the governing category; the presence of Infl is sufficient. They therefore propose to replace the term "subject" with "Infl" in the definition, as in (15) (their (9)).

(15) γ is a governing category for α iff
γ is the minimal category that contains α and a governor for α and has an Infl.

This definition, which embodies a broader notion of governing category, now accounts for the Italian data. Yet as Manzini and Wexler show, even this is not enough. The Icelandic reflexive *sig* violates the Binding Conditions, even under the new definition. ((16a–d) are Manzini and Wexler's (10)–(13).)

(16) a. Jón$_j$ segir að Maria$_i$ elskar sig$_{i/*j}$
Jón says that Maria loves Refl
b. Jón$_j$ segir að   Maria$_i$ elski   sig$_{i/j}$
Jón says that Maria loves(subjunctive) Refl
c. Maria$_j$ skipaði Haraldi$_i$ að PRO raka   sig$_{i/j}$
Maria ordered Harald   to   shave Refl
d. Jón$_i$ heyrði lysingu   Mariu$_i$ af ser$_{i/j}$
Jón heard description Maria(gen) of Refl
'Jón heard Maria's description of Refl.'

To account for these data, a new, still more inclusive definition of governing category is needed. Manzini and Wexler propose the definition in (17) (their (14)).

(17) γ is a governing category for α iff
γ is the minimal category that contains α and a governor for α and has a "referential" Tense.

By "referential" Tense they mean a tense that has inherently defined properties, rather than an "anaphoric" Tense—that is, one whose properties depend on some superordinate Tense. Now the data in (16) are accounted for.

Icelandic, however, poses further problems. The pronominal *hann* violates the Binding Conditions in certain instances, even under definition (17) of governing category. ((18a–c) are Manzini and Wexler's (15)–(17).)

(18) a. Jón$_i$ segir að   Maria elskar hann$_i$
       Jón says that Maria loves him

    b. Jón$_i$ segir að   Maria elski   hann$_i$.
       Jón says that Maria loves (subjunctive) him

    c. *Jón$_i$ skipaði mér að raka   hann$_i$.
       Jón ordered me to shave him

By the above definitions, the governing category for *hann* is the embedded sentence in all the cases in (18). Binding Condition B predicts that *hann* must be free in the embedded sentence, thus correctly predicting the grammaticality of (18a–b) but incorrectly predicting that (18c) will also be grammatical. Thus, Manzini and Wexler propose another modification of the definition of governing category (their (18)).

(19) γ is a governing category for α iff
    γ is the minimal category that contains α and a governor for α and has a Tense.

But even this is not sufficient to account for the variation the world's languages exhibit with respect to governing categories. The Japanese anaphor *zibun* requires further modifications. ((20a–b) are Manzini and Wexler's (19)–(20).)

(20) a. John-wa$_j$ [Bill-ga$_i$ zibun-o$_{i/j}$ nikunde iru] to   omotte iru.
       John   Bill   Refl   hates   that thinks
       'John thinks that Bill hates Refl.'

    b. John-wa$_j$ [Bill-ga$_i$ zibun-no$_{i/j}$ syasin-o mihatte iru] to   omotte iru.
       John   Bill   Refl   pictures is watching that thinks
       'John thinks that Bill is watching pictures of Refl.'

These sentences violate the Binding Conditions under any of the above definitions. Thus, Manzini and Wexler propose a still more inclusive definition of governing category (their (21)).

(21) γ is a governing category for α iff
    γ is the minimal category that contains α and a governor for α and has a "root" Tense.

With five different definitions of governing category—(13), (15), (17), (19), (21)—we are now ready for a parametric definition of governing category (Manzini and Wexler's (22)).

(22) γ is a governing category for α iff
    γ is the minimal category that contains α and a governor for α and has
    a. a subject; or
    b. an Infl; or
    c. a Tense; or
    d. a "referential" Tense; or
    e. a "root" Tense.

Now Manzini and Wexler derive the most important property of this parametric definition. The values of the parameter are ordered with respect to one another in the inclusion relation; that is, the language defined if we choose the value in (22a) is a proper subset of the language defined by (22b), and so on. In so doing, Manzini and Wexler present a perfect case of the application of the Subset Principle.

From the point of view of language learning, we can see how the Subset Principle interacts with the parameter system. As part of their inborn language faculty, children have the Binding Conditions, with their five-valued parametric formulation of governing category. No theory of markedness is necessary, because the Subset Principle will determine, on the basis of the input, what value will be fixed. Thus, the Subset Principle characterizes a sequence of five grammars ordered as in (22). Notice that although the parametric values are stated in the grammar without order, the order in the sequence S is fixed due to the Subset Principle. Children, then, begin with the assumption that they are speakers of English, and, upon being confronted with evidence to the contrary, they move on from subset to superset, until they converge on the actual grammar of their mother tongue.

As we can see, then, extremely interesting predictions come out of the interaction between the Subset Principle and the Regression Hypothesis when applied to the parametric definition of binding.

6.3.4   The Dissolution-Acquisition Interaction

The interaction between the Subset Principle and the Regression Hypothesis also has interesting consequences for the relation between language acquisition and language dissolution. Generally, the sequence of aphasic grammars S' turns out to be the mirror image of the child's sequence S, because that is what the Regression Hypothesis requires.

Given this requirement, the set relation that holds between successive members of the sequence S' is clear: the sequence of aphasic grammars must meet the *inverse* of the Subset Principle, which we may call the *Superset Principle*. To state this formally, if (1) for every pair in sequence S, G_i, G_{i+1}, $L(G_i) \subseteq L(G_{i+1})$ by the Subset Principle, and (2) S' is ordered inversely to S by the Regression Hypothesis, then the principle in (23) holds.

(23) *Superset Principle*
    In the sequence $S' = G'_1,...,G'_n$, for every $1 \leq i \leq n$
    $L(G'_i) \supseteq L(G'_{i+1})$.

Thus, the relation between two succeeding grammars in S' is again that of proper inclusion, yet S and S' proceed in opposite directions.

We can summarize this discussion in the claim shown in (24).

(24) If the Regression Hypothesis (1) and the Subset Principle (9) are true, then the Superset Principle (23) must be true.

Now it is time to examine the three definitions of aphasic grammar given in (2), to see whether the Regression Hypothesis can be constructed coherently under any of them. These definitions are repeated in (25).

(25) The notion "aphasic grammar" will be interpreted as follows:
    a. For every G'_j, $1 \leq j \leq n$, in (1) there is an aphasic syndrome, and for every syndrome there is a G'_j.
    b. For every G'_j, $1 \leq j \leq n$, in (1) there is a stage of recovery in a given aphasic syndrome, and for every such stage there is a G'_j.
    c. For every G'_j, $1 \leq j \leq n$, in (1) there is a degree of severity in a given aphasic syndrome, and for every such degree there is a G'_j.

A second property of the sequence S' concerns the relation between the aphasic and the normal language. The first grammar in the sequence S' (namely, G'_1) is the normal grammar. It thus follows, by (23), that for every other aphasic grammar G'_i, $1 \leq i \leq n$, $L(G'_i) \subseteq L(G'_1)$. The aphasic language, then, can never be larger than the normal language in the domain of the Subset Principle. That is, in this domain no ungrammatical sentence can be generated by the aphasic grammar.

Finally, it is predicted that for every stage in acquisition there is a corresponding aphasic grammar, and vice versa.

The Regression Hypothesis in the sense of (25a) would be construed as meaning that for every stage in acquisition there is an aphasic syndrome, and vice versa. Adding the considerations that follow from the Subset Principle leads to the notion that the languages defined by these syndromes stand in a relation of proper inclusion to one another. This means that the grammars representing the various aphasic syndromes are ordered in such a way that each generates a language that is a subset of the preceding one. Importantly, since the order is not given a priori, the Regression Hypothesis is vacuous. In addition, this view of aphasia is incompatible with any position found in the literature. Most authors (and notably Jakobson) tend to think that the different syndromes stand in complementary distribution to one another, rather than in an inclusion relation. This is because complementary distribution implies that their intersection is empty. Therefore, even authors who have applied the Regression Hypothesis to syndromes—for instance, Wepman and Jones (1964)—would probably not support this view once it is spelled out. We can thus rule out construing the Regression Hypothesis in the sense of (25a).

Next let us try construing the hypothesis in the sense of (25b), which says that the stages of recovery in any aphasic syndrome correspond to the stages of acquisition, yet in inverse order. Unlike the previous interpretation of the notion "aphasic grammar," this one offers a strong empirical hypothesis for evaluation. It is quite unlikely that *all* aphasic syndromes will exhibit this effect, because they are so different in form from one another, yet some of them might.

But what theory of recovery is necessary for the Regression Hypothesis to be true under this interpretation? The hypothesis is very strong in that it requires not just the same number of stages in acquisition and recovery, but also the same stages. Therefore, the theory of recovery must be parametrized, and it will now have to specify the parameters that are (re)fixed during recovery. This means that the aphasic must be sensitive to positive evidence—yet we have seen that such a possibility is quite implausible.

We are therefore left with construing the Regression Hypothesis according to the definition in (25c). This is perhaps its most widely held interpretation, namely, that aphasic syndromes exhibit degrees of severity that mimic stages of acquisition. The claim stated in (24) would then be that languages generated by successive grammars have to stand in a proper inclusion relation to one another—in other words, the more severe the impairment, the smaller the language generated by the aphasic's grammar. This hypothesis is compatible with the view, close to that expressed by Ribot's Law, that the later an element (or construction, or rule) is acquired, the more susceptible it is to impairment. That is, the more severe the impairment, the farther the aphasic's language is from the final state, and the closer it is to the initial state. This is a consequence of the Superset Principle. On this view, which is more or less the one taken by Hyams (1986b), aphasic impairment is "unlearning" language.

What is most interesting about the claim under consideration (that is, (24) with (1) interpreted in the sense of (2c)) is that it provides a formalism whose empirical adequacy can be tested along various lines. Most important, it has the property that for any degree of impairment, an aphasic grammar can *never* generate a language that is a superset of the patient's previous, normal language, that the aphasic grammar must be a possible grammar, and that it must be one of those attested for children. It also provides a severity metric: the smaller the language is, the more severe the aphasia. The validity of this metric can be investigated experimentally and compared to other, nonlinguistic measures, such as lesion size and locus, fluency, time post onset, and so on. Yet we must bear in mind that these considerations hold only for the domain of the Subset Principle. The claims from which this discussion follows depend crucially on the Subset Principle as a theory of learning (whose domain is restricted by the Subset Condition) and on a particular version of the Regression Hypothesis.

In sum, the interaction of the Regression Hypothesis (construed in terms of a syndrome's degree of severity) and the Subset Principle provides an empirical claim that has testable consequences.

(26) If the Regression Hypothesis (construed in the sense of (25c)) and the Subset Principle are true, then, in the domain of the latter,

   a. The aphasic language is always a subset of the normal language.
   b. Degrees of severity are expressible in terms of proper inclusion relations of the respective aphasic languages (Superset Principle).
   c. The languages observed for aphasics must correspond to intermediate stages observed in acquisition, and vice versa.

6.3.5 Predictions

What implications do these claims have for binding in aphasia? If the governing category parameter is true, then several things follow. Consider, first of all, Japanese-speaking aphasics. According to Manzini and Wexler, their language is the largest with respect to binding. Therefore, the Regression Hypothesis predicts that there is a class of Japanese-speaking aphasics corresponding to each of the five possible values of the governing category parameter. According to this claim, then, there are Japanese-speaking aphasics who exhibit Icelandic binding effects, Japanese-speaking aphasics who exhibit Italian binding effects, and Japanese-speaking aphasics who exhibit English binding effects.[4]

Next consider Italian-speaking aphasics. The Regression Hypothesis predicts that they might exhibit English binding effects. Crucially, however, they may never have Icelandic or Japanese definitions of governing category, because the languages generated under these definitions are larger than Italian, violating the Superset Principle. Similarly, Icelandic-speaking aphasics may exhibit Italian or English binding effects, but not Japanese. Finally, English-speaking aphasics cannot adopt any of the other values of the governing category parameter, because any change would result in a violation of the Superset Principle.

Some examples are now in order. Breakdown in the use of anaphors will always move in the direction of the smaller language. For the languages in question, then, the order would be Japanese > Icelandic > Italian > English. No aphasic can violate Binding Condition A by extending the definition of governing category, and thus English-speaking aphasics cannot violate this condition at all. For Italian-speaking aphasics, however, violations in the opposite direction (adopting the English definition of governing category even when it is not permitted) are predicted. For these aphasics, then, sentences like (27a–b) would no longer be grammatical, even though they are for the normal speaker of Italian.

(27) a. Alice$_i$ vide Mario$_j$ guardare sè$_i$ nello specchio.
     Alice   saw Mario   look at   Refl in the mirror
   b. Alice$_i$ guardò   i ritratti di sè$_i$ di Mario$_j$.
     Alice   looked at portraits of Refl of Mario
   'Alice looked at Mario's portraits of Refl.'

It is predicted, then, that under no circumstances will Italian-speaking aphasics adopt the interpretation of these sentences on which *sè* is coindexed with *Alice*. Instead, they will always interpret (27a) in such a way that *Mario* looks at himself only, and never at *Alice*, even though the other interpretation is normally possible in Italian. Similarly, these patients will always interpret the portraits in (27b) to be portraits of Mario and not of Alice, although in Italian both interpretations are possible.

Similar considerations hold for Icelandic and Japanese. For normal speakers of Icelandic (28) is grammatical, but for Icelandic-speaking aphasics it is predicted to be ungrammatical.

(28) Jon$_i$ segir að   Maria elskar hann$_i$.
    Jon says that Maria loves   him

In Japanese the same type of prediction would hold for (29a–b).

(29) a. John-wa$_j$ [Bill-ga$_i$ zibun-o$_{i/j}$ nikunde iru] to   omotte iru.
       John   Bill   Refl   hates   that thinks
     'John thinks that Bill hates Refl.'
   b. John-wa$_j$ [Bill-ga$_i$ zibun-no$_{i/j}$ syasin-o mihatte iru] to   omotte iru
     John   Bill   Refl   pictures is watching that thinks
     'John thinks that Bill is watching pictures of Refl.'

These are only some of the available predictions. With respect to binding theory, all the cases Manzini and Wexler consider as counterexamples to the standard definition of governing category (to which the Subset Principle applies) are predicted to be ungrammatical for aphasics who abide by the Superset Principle. With respect to pronouns, the predictions are precisely reversed.

With respect to degrees of severity, we can also derive the prediction that among Japanese-speaking aphasics we will find severely impaired patients who exhibit English binding patterns, less severely impaired patients who exhibit Italian binding patterns, even less severely impaired patients who exhibit Icelandic binding patterns, and so on. The Superset Principle provides a clear framework within which to evaluate severity in aphasia—assuming, of course, that the Subset Principle and the Regression Hypothesis are valid.

Yet there is a third prediction, which is perhaps easier to assess experimentally—namely, that the aphasic language may never exceed the normal one in the intended sense. This we can test by examining the aphasic grammar to see whether it generates ungrammatical strings in the relevant domain. In the case of English anaphora we would predict that any binding violation that follows from the extension of the definition of governing category would be detected. For example, aphasics should always construe the anaphors in (30) as referring to *Bill*, never to *John*, just as normal speakers do.

(30) John told Bill to wash himself.

We are thus able to make very strong predictions concerning the cross-linguistic impairment of grammatical abilities in aphasia. We also have a severity metric. The Regression Hypothesis predicts, first, that the smaller the language generated by a particular choice of parametric value, the less prone the parameter should be to impairment. In the previous example, then, English is less susceptible to impairment of binding than Italian, Icelandic, and Japanese. Second, the hypothesis predicts that for every observed stage of acquisition, there is a corresponding degree of severity in aphasia. Empirical evidence bearing on this issue is naturally hard to come by, but there are some hints. In the next section we will examine these two predictions in light of the available empirical evidence.

6.3.6   Empirical Evidence: Acquisition versus Breakdown

To date none of the three empirical claims that follow from the Superset Principle as stated has been tested directly. However, bits of evidence can be gathered from the literature and brought to bear on the issues in question. Although there is a substantial body of relevant data on the development of binding relations (see Crain and McKee 1986; Jakubowicz 1984; Lust 1986; Solan 1983; Wexler and Chien 1985, 1988), there is very little experimental evidence on language breakdown. Although the available evidence is far from systematic, some preliminary clues can be extracted from past experimentation. Specifically, three studies are relevant: those carried out by Blumstein et al. (1983), Crain and Shankweiler (1985), and Grodzinsky et al. (1989). Here we will investigate two implications of the Superset Principle empirically. First, we will compare the development of reflexives to their breakdown. Second, we will look at the claim that aphasics may never have a grammar that generates a language larger than normal with respect to binding principles (or more precisely, the definition of governing category).

Consider first the findings reported by Wexler and Chien (1988). They conducted an extensive longitudinal study to assess the development of Binding Conditions A and B and to determine whether acquisition data can decide a theoretical debate between competing approaches to binding, a debate whose essentials have been discussed in chapter 4.

Wexler and Chien's experiment includes several conditions, many of which (especially those involving quantified NP anaphora) bear directly on the formulation of binding theory. Here, though, we will concentrate on aspects of the experiment that are relevant to the acquisition-dissolution comparison. This experiment was a follow-up to a previous one in which Wexler and Chien had already found differences between pronouns and anaphors in children's comprehension. This time, though, they tested Reinhart's theory against the standard GB view, as presented in chapters 2 and 4.

Their experiment consisted of a sentence-verification task that tested various structures involving pronouns and reflexives with various antecedents. It included six conditions.

(31) a. Is Mama Bear touching herself?
 b. Is Mama Bear touching her?
 c. Is every bear touching herself?
 d. Is every bear touching her?
 e. Is Mama Bear touching Donald Duck?
 f. Is every bear touching Donald Duck?

Children saw one picture and heard one sentence at a time, and they were supposed to say "yes" if the sentence accurately described the picture and "no" if it did not. In each condition there were 12 sentences, half requiring a positive answer and half a negative answer. The pictures showed a cartoon character performing some action either on itself or on another.

Wexler and Chien found that only on (31b) did the children perform poorly— even the older groups remained at chance levels. In all the other conditions the children quickly developed abilities that brought them to performance levels above chance, indicating good comprehension of the structure involved.

The same experiment (alluded to in chapter 4) has been administered to agrammatic aphasics, whose performance was virtually identical to that of the children (Grodzinsky et al., 1989).

What do these findings imply about the development-breakdown issue? Notice first that they do not bear directly on the governing category question, which is the one for which we have assumed the Subset Principle applies. Notice also that all we are looking at is a single syndrome, not differentiated for degrees of severity, which the Superset Principle would require, so all we have is a snapshot of one of the grammars in the sequence S' of impaired grammars. But since we have evidence from different stages of acquisition, the comparison is instructive.

Do these findings comport with the Regression Hypothesis? Given the paucity of data, the question can be answered only conditionally at the moment: if the constructions in question are within the scope of the Subset Principle, then the Regression Hypothesis is supported. Since the Regression Hypothesis is the claim that aphasia is acquisition in reverse, the breakdown of language can never exhibit aberrant performance patterns that are not attested in development. If so, then the present comparison provides evidence in this direction. Following Noam Chomsky's suggestion given in chapter 4, one could say that a principle that forces the generalization of Binding Condition B, which is initially stated for bound pronouns only, develops over time in the growing child and is lost in aphasia, thus confirming the Regression Hypothesis.

It is not clear, however, that what children acquire (and aphasics lose) is Binding Condition B. As shown in chapter 4, the data favor Reinhart's construal of binding theory—that is, that the children and the aphasics are deficient with respect to Reinhart's inference rule, not the Binding Conditions. This rule is thus acquired and then lost. Whether or not it is under the scope of the Regression Hypothesis is an open question.

Next consider the Superset Principle and its implications concerning the relative size of the aphasic and normal languages—namely, that the former can never be larger than the latter. This is so because, by the Regression Hypothesis, every aphasic grammar has a developing counterpart, and, by the Subset Principle, there is no child grammar that generates a language larger than the adult language (in the domain of the Subset Principle, that is). If so, then aphasics should never generate any ungrammatical strings in the relevant domain. For instance, aphasics should never exhibit errors that are due to the binding of an anaphor by an antecedent outside the governing category, because this would imply that the grammar is based on a definition of governing category that generates a language that is larger than normal. Again, this is not what is found.

Crain and Shankweiler (1985) conducted a grammaticality judgment experiment with agrammatic aphasics. In one case at least they found that the subjects systematically coindexed the reflexive with an antecedent that was outside the governing category, as shown in (32).

(32) a. *John threatened Mary to spray bug-spray on herself.

   b. John$_i$ threatened Mary$_j$ [$_{gc}$PRO$_i$ to spray bug-spray on Refl$_{i/*j}$]

As we can see from (32b), the definition of governing category must be changed and extended for sentences like (32a) to be judged grammatical; in other words, the reflexive must be bound to *Mary,* which is outside the governing category. Indeed, the agrammatic aphasics incorrectly judged this sentence grammatical 75 percent of the time, which indicated systematic error (below chance). This performance cannot be due to errors in gender, because in conditions that involved other syntactic constructions the patients performed correctly when gender was the only clue to grammaticality. Crain and Shankweiler correctly point out that the finding might indicate that "agrammatic aphasics tend to adopt a minimal distance strategy when confronted with special syntactic complexities."[5] But reasons for error aside, the patients clearly exhibited performance that is governed by an abnormal grammatical system. In particular, this system generates a language that is larger than normal, contrary to what the Superset Principle would predict. Thus, even though the available evidence is not systematic and is open to more than one interpretation, there are already some preliminary clues pointing to the validity of the Regression Hypothesis. Obviously, direct tests should be devised, to adduce more compelling evidence.

6.4   Conclusion

Taking a century-old claim seriously, and recasting it in current terminology and conception, may be worthwhile at times. We have seen that an explicit formulation of the Regression Hypothesis has consequences and yields interesting predictions that can be tested experimentally. A preliminary requirement for the statement of this hypothesis is a coherent learning theory. Once such a theory is assumed, the hypothesis can be formally stated, and clear predictions follow. The available evidence does not support the hypothesis, yet because of its scattered nature it does not provide a compelling enough basis for rejecting it, either. What is needed now is a systematic investigation of the hypothesis, across languages and across varying degrees of severity of each aphasic syndrome. This investigation is important because it might offer clues about the relation between the way things are learned and their arrangement in the central nervous system. Language learning and the functional arrangement of the language faculty can be related in any number of ways, starting with an arbitrary relation, through a relation according to which the first item learned is the first to be impaired, to a relation defined by the Regression Hypothesis. There is something intuitive about this last relation, but it need not hold. Thus, if the relation between the learning and dissolution of language is other than arbitrary, then what is learned must be subject to severe constraints: grammar (or aspects thereof) must now have the property that it is learned and "unlearned" in a manner defined by the relation that is found to hold (according to the Regression Hypothesis or whatever).

There are more reasons why the Regression Hypothesis and other conceivable nonarbitrary relations between language acquisition and language breakdown are interesting theoretically. Should evidence supporting any of them be found, several claims will receive indirect empirical support. First, the learning theory that is assumed will immediately be fortified. The learning theory assumed here is not logically necessary; rather, the motivation for it is empirical. Thus, evidence supporting the Regression Hypothesis will indirectly support the learning theory. Second, if cross-linguistic patterns of impairment are found to be as predicted, then the linguistic analysis of the relevant constructions—in the present case Manzini and Wexler's parametric account—will also be strengthened. And although we have pursued the consequences of just one version of the Regression Hypothesis and the learning strategy, other versions are possible. For the moment everything is vastly underdetermined by the available data. Thus, this discussion is just a demonstration of how one can approach the two related areas, and it is certainly not intended to be the final word.

Notes

Chapter 1

1. See, in this respect, work done by Farah (1985) on mental imagery and by Etcoff (1984) on face recognition and the perception of affect. See also some hints in Marr's (1982) work, concerning object recognition.

2. See, for example, Berndt and Caramazza 1980, concerning language deficits; Caramazza and McCloskey 1985, concerning acalculia; and Kolk and van Grunsven 1985, concerning agrammatism.

3. For collections of papers representing this view of linguistics and psycholinguistics, see Joos 1954 and Osgood and Sebeok 1954, respectively.

4. This, despite the fact that it was recognized that at least some syndromes involved selective impairment to some linguistic elements but not others. These observations were never seen as significant. See chapter 3 and Pick 1913.

5. Another, "mixed" approach should be mentioned, a good representative of which is presented by Zaidel and Schweiger (1983). "Mixed" models use terms borrowed from information-processing theory and localize them in the two cerebral hemispheres. The functional architecture of the system is thus equated with the actual layout of the brain. This approach takes notions like "pathway" and "processor" from processing models, which are used there to denote functional connections among processing constituents, and seeks to identify them with fiber bundles and areas of the brain. It is thus a hybrid between connectionism and information processing and hence seems to suffer from every drawback of each.

6. There are actually some exceptions in this respect. Kimura (1976) has claimed that linguistic activities are but an extension of the motor system and that all language impairments can be explained in motor-theoretic terms. Earlier Schuell (1965) claimed that Broca's aphasia is actually an "apraxia for speech." However, such approaches deny a wide variety of facts. For example, no conceivable motor theory can account for the differential treatment that agrammatic aphasics give different syntactic constructions or vocabulary types. The description of these deficits must make reference to *grammatical* terms. This approach, then, cannot be taken too seriously.

7. However, an increasing number of studies have investigated other performances, most notably, the time-course of language comprehension. See Bradley, Garrett, and Zurif 1980; Swinney et al. 1985; and the references to follow in the text.

8. One exception is the use of drugs. For instance, in the well-known sodium amytal technique, subjects receive an intracarotid injection of a substance that temporarily blocks an entire hemisphere. See Wada and Rasmussen 1960.

Chapter 2

1. For elaboration, see the following sources: Lightfoot 1983 and Chomsky 1988 provide a general introduction to modern linguistics; Akmajian and Heny 1975 is a syntax primer; Van Riemsdijk and Williams 1986, Sells 1986, and Lasnik and Uriagereka 1988 are advanced texts on current developments.

2. It should be noted that at least some of these statements cover up hotly debated issues, which are beyond the scope of this introduction.

Chapter 3

1. According to Mohr (1976), the area relevant to the signs observed in Broca's aphasia is larger than Broca originally thought. It may involve all the area supplied by the upper division of the middle cerebral artery and its tributaries, ranging from the operculum anteriorly, through Broca's area, to anterior parietal regions, insula, both banks of the central (Rolandic) fissure, usually extending deep into the hemisphere.

2. It could be either an incomplete word, which simply needs an additional piece of morphology, or an abstract word, such as those discussed in the introductory chapter to Chomsky 1955/1975 in connection with Hebrew word structure.

3. Kean (1977) offers predictions for languages other than English. One is that Russian-speaking agrammatic patients would always speak in nominative masculine nouns, because they provide a zero-inflection option. Yet many nouns in this language have overt nominatives and no zero-form. Kean's prediction is that patients would produce only stems for these nouns, which is obviously false.

4. This utterance, like the others in the 1973 English translation of Panse and Shimoyama, is given without context, so it is hard to determine why the tense is wrong.

5. Also, under a view that the deficit in production parallels the deficit in comprehension, agrammatic patients are predicted to accept sentences containing substitutions of inflectional features. There is some empirical evidence to that effect, coming from grammaticality judgment experiments. See Grossman and Haberman 1982; Gardner, Denes, and Zurif 1975; Linebarger, Schwartz, and Saffran 1983; Zurif and Grodzinsky 1983.

6. Bates et al. (1986) claim that, contrary to the prediction made here, substitutions of agrammatic aphasics are always off the mark by at most one feature. If true, this would require further restriction of the present proposal. The data, however, seem to me so impoverished that a clear case cannot be made either way.

7. The account in Grodzinsky 1984a states, roughly, that features are deleted at S-structure. However, it also stipulates a default mechanism: namely, that whenever a word has a zero-inflection option, agrammatics will choose this option. This clearly unmotivated stipulation was invoked to account for the fact that agrammatic speakers of English-like languages tend to omit inflections, whereas agrammatic speakers of Hebrew-like languages tend to subsitute. We have seen, however, that there is no need for such a mechanism, because the correct results are forced by the interaction between (4) and the preserved principles of grammar.

8. Stephen Crain (personal communication) points out that not every element that occupies a determiner position is impaired in agrammatism. Specifically, *Mary* is in determiner position in NPs like *Mary's hat*, yet it is not omitted (or substituted) in agrammatic speech. The statement in (8) does not exclude such elements, however. The structure of the NPs in question is shown in (i).

(i)

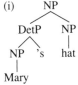

Thus, this account predicts that *Mary*, being a terminal immediately dominated by a lexical category, will be preserved and that the possessive s will be omitted, which is precisely what Goodglass and Hunt (1958) and others report. Thus, (8) predicts the data correctly. In fact, if the proposal made in the text is to be extended to comprehension, then there is some corroborating evidence from a study of the comprehension of quantificational NPs by agrammatic aphasics, presented by Shapiro et al. (1986). Such an extension runs into empirical difficulties, however; findings by Lukatela, Crain, and Shankweiler (1988) regarding Serbo-Croatian-speaking agrammatics' appreciation of case relations, as attested by their performance in grammaticality judgment, speak directly against it.

9. This prediction contrasts with Kean's. According to her account, some derivational morphemes (such as *-ness* in *sadness*) will be omitted, and others (such as *-ity* in *continuity*) will be retained.

10. There are two exceptions to this: Goodglass (1968) reports an experiment that reveals a comprehension disorder in agrammatism, and Parisi and Pizzamiglio (1970) report a similar finding. For a review of earlier work, see Goodglass 1976. Goodglass notes that a comprehension deficit in agrammatism was pointed out by Pick and Goldstein, among others, even though no one attempted an accurate characterization.

11. Other studies have examined the processing abilities in agrammatism, yet most of them focus on aspects of this syndrome that are not relevant here. See Zurif, Swinney, and Garrett (in press) for a recent review.

12. See Zurif and Grodzinsky 1983 for a reinterpretation of these findings in terms of the proposal made in Grodzinsky 1984a.

13. In this task a third picture is presented: a lexical distractor that can be ignored for the present discussion.

14. If one wished to advance a claim that correlates impairment of function with lesion site, then it would be weakened due to the inconclusiveness expressed in the text. But I make no such claim here; my perspective is purely functional.

15. Some investigators have claimed that agrammatic patients are unstable, that there is variation even within the same patient (Badecker and Caramazza 1985; Kolk and van Grunsven 1985b). If these claims are correct, then neuropsychological research of the form espoused here should be abandoned. It seems to me, however, that these claims are false, as attested by the converging evidence from many laboratories that is reviewed

below. To the extent that there is some apparent variability in the data, it is due either to poorly controlled experiments or to incoherent interpretation of findings. It is important to note, though, that from the perspective of these authors, the fact that all these data can be accounted for uniformly, by a single generalization, is purely accidental—nothing short of a miracle. A detailed examination of this claim is beyond the scope of this book; but see, for example, Grodzinsky and Marek 1988.

16. Pictures shown to subjects in the experiments always depicted the content of the relative clause, not the main clause.

17. Throughout the discussion I have been assuming a framework that admits string-vacuous movement. As a result, there have been traces in subject position of relative clauses, bringing the Default Principle into action in these cases. This analysis is quite controversial (for conflicting views, see Ross 1967; Clements et al. 1983; Chomsky 1986b). Whatever the correct analysis may be, however, it is orthogonal to the account of agrammatism. This is because the analyses make overlapping predictions for agrammatic comprehension, which are actually borne out. If vacuous movement is assumed, then the Default Principle assigns the role of agent correctly, and patients are expected to perform at above-chance level on these sentences. If vacuous movement is not assumed, then nothing is deleted from the representations of subject relatives, and patients again are expected to perform correctly.

18. These belong to the subclass of subject-experiencer verbs and are thus distinct from verbs of the object-experiencer subclass, such as *bother*. See Johnson 1985, Belletti and Rizzi 1988, Pesetsky 1987, and the discussion that follows.

19. In principle, then, even for simple agentive actives there could be a pathology that assigns, say, the role of location to the subject and the role of theme to the object, and under our assumptions the patients' performance would still be indistinguishable from that of normal speakers.

20. One objection, raised by Hagit Borer, is that the notion of agentive psychological verbs is semantically incoherent. Thus, semantic coherence must be checked not just at the level of a single item but also at the clausal level. Yet as Barry Schein notes, we must recall the situation in which patients respond. They have a forced-choice task: they are told, in this case, to order cards in a way that matches a picture. Given that they must use the strategy, they will pick the most salient actor and assign the NP corresponding to it the highest role in the Thematic Hierarchy (in this case, agent). This will result in below-chance performance, for the reasons specified in the text.

21. Steven Pinker has pointed out another potential problem facing this account: if the thematic representation of a sentence contains (say) two instruments, then it has no theme (or stimulus) role, and again the representation is potentially incoherent semantically. Still, patients can use the little they have—namely, the information that subject = agent—and give a consistently wrong response. Thus, although the thematic representation may be incoherent for the patients, consistent inversion is the only response they will give if forced to give some response. But notice that almost all of these verbs have an object-experiencer counterpart: *fear/frighten, see/show, enjoy/please,* and so on. Although the overlap is not perfect, and each class contains verbs that do not have a counterpart in the other (for example, *know, surprise*), it is tempting to assume that the members of each subject-agent/object-experiencer pair both have the same lexical entry, except that one is

the mirror image of the other. Once we make such an assumption, we can say that the aphasic interprets passivized verbs of the first group as if they were active verbs of the second.

22. The constructions in (52), and some others, are currently being tested in an experiment designed and carried out by Amy Pierce.

Concerning (52d): If this construction were to yield chance performance, contrary to what is predicted, we would have to reformulate the account. Specifically, we would be forced to assume that implicit arguments, such as the agent in agentless passives, are represented thematically and hence are there to create a conflict with the strategy. This in fact agrees with current analyses of passivization proposed in generative grammar (Jaeggli 1986, 614; Baker, Johnson, and Roberts 1989).

Concerning (52e): See note 17 with respect to vacuous movement.

23. We would not be alone in making this move. In fact, many proposals to account for normal language violate Lasnik and Kupin's formalism. For example, May (1985) points out that adjunction structures like (i) violate the X' schema (which requires a one-to-one relation between X^0 and its projections) in that more than one XP dominates X^0.

(i)

To solve this problem, May proposes that one category dominates another iff all the *segments* of the first dominate the second. Note where this proposal leads, however: YP in (i) cannot be dominated by XP, because there is a segment of XP that does not dominate YP. But YP also does not dominate XP. It follows, as Speas (1986) points out, that neither precedence nor dominance relations hold between XP and YP. Since according to Lasnik and Kupin's model, one of these relations must hold between every two nodes of a well-formed tree, May's theory also violates their formalism.

Chapter 4

1. Some, in fact, have claimed that grammatical intuitions are not the right kind of data for theories that account for our linguistic performance. See, for example, Bever 1970.

2. Notice that not every issue in linguistics can be resolved by reference to breakdown patterns, since there is no logical necessity for any breakdown pattern to exist.

3. However, it remains to be demonstrated exactly how one can predict theta-role reversal with psychological passives and chance performance on agentive passives by assuming either GPSG or LFG as the descriptive framework.

4. A reviewer inquires why another type of adjectival passive—namely, *-able* adjectives, as in *This book is readable*—was not tested. The reason is that it is impossible to construct examples that have the necessary "semantic reversibility" property and contain an adjective that is relatively frequent in the language. These two properties are essential if a meaningful test of agrammatic aphasics is to be conducted, especially given the available subject population, most of whom are patients at Veterans Administration hospitals. We have in fact attempted to test this construction, so far unsuccessfully.

5. Preliminary findings from Hebrew indicate that agrammatic patients cannot coindex resumptive pronouns. In constructions such as *ha-yeled she-ha-' ish daxaf 'oto hu shamen* `the boy who the man pushed HIM was fat', the patients perform no better than they do on the transformationally derived analogous relative clause (the same but without the pronoun). This runs contrary to the Trace-Deletion Hypothesis, which claims that the impairment is restricted to movement. However, a generalization over the impaired pronouns and resumptives is possible.

Chapter 5

1. See Bruner 1973 for a representative collection of articles, regarding theoretical as well as empirical issues.

2. See, for example, Marslen-Wilson and Tyler 1980, Anderson 1983, Simon 1969, Schank 1973, and Rumelhart and McClelland 1986.

3. Because one of the properties of Fodor's modules is speed, it is commonly believed that the evidence most relevant to modularity comes from the time-course of processing. There are reasons to believe, however, that modules are not necessarily fast. Chomsky (1986a) gives examples of sentences that cannot be computed quickly. Similarly, Julesz (1971) has provided evidence that visual recognition may require long times if the right stimulus is chosen. Yet even if modules are taken to be mandatorily fast, it is still not logically necessary that the only relevant information about them should come from reaction time.

Chapter 6

1. Along with many others, such as Pinker (1984), Hyams makes the additional assumption that language learning is not instantaneous, as Chomsky (1965) assumes. That is, there are observable stages in the development of language that reflect particular mental states of the child—in other words, that reflect the child's having an incomplete grammatical system compared to the adult. See Borer and Wexler (1986) for further discussion of this issue.

2. By sensitivity to such data I do not mean local correction, namely, reuttering of a particular word, phrase, or sentence. Rather, I mean a correction that reflects the acquisition of an internalized rule.

3. In fact, Hyams's claims are compatible with Ribot's Law more than with Jakobson's claims, because only Ribot's Law explicitly mentions susceptibility to impairment as a function of acquisition time. Jakobson's claims touch only on the relation between the observed arrangements of sequences—that stages of language learning mirror stages of language loss.

4. This may be true only under a very strong version of Independence; see Manzini and Wexler 1987.

5. This characterization should actually be refined to refer to overt grammatical categories only.

References

Akmajian, A., and F. Heny (1975). *An introduction to the principles of transformational syntax.* Cambridge, MA: MIT Press.

Anderson, J. R. (1983). *The architecture of cognition.* Cambridge, MA: Harvard University Press.

Ansell, B., and C. Flowers (1982). Aphasic adults' use of heuristic and structural linguistic cues for analysis. *Brain and Language* 16, 61–72.

Badecker, W., and A. Caramazza (1985). On considerations of method and theory governing the use of clinical categories in neurolinguistics and cognitive neuropsychology: The case against agrammatism. *Cognition* 20, 97–126.

Baker, C. L. (1979). Syntactic theory and the projection problem. *Linguistic Inquiry* 10, 533–581.

Baker, M., K. Johnson, and I. Roberts (1989). Passive arguments raised. *Linguistic Inquiry* 20, 219–251.

Bates, E., A. Friederici, G. Miceli, and B. Wulfeck (1986). Comprehension in aphasia: A cross-linguistic study. Ms., UCSD, Max Planck Institute and Catholic University, Rome.

Belletti, A., and L. Rizzi (1988). Psych-verbs and th-theory. *Natural Language and Linguistic Theory* 6, 291–352.

Benson, D. F. (1979). Aphasia. In K. Heilman and E. Valenstein, eds., *Clinical Neuropsychology.* New York: Oxford University Press.

Berndt, R. S., and A. Caramazza (1980). A redefinition of the syndrome of Broca's aphasia: Implications for a neuropsychological model of language. *Applied Psycholinguistics* 1, 225–278.

Berwick, R. (1982). Locality principles and the acquisition of syntactic knowledge. Doctoral dissertation, MIT.

Berwick, R., and A. Weinberg (1984). *The grammatical basis of linguistic performance.* Cambridge, MA: MIT Press.

Berwick R., and A. Weinberg (1985). Deterministic parsing and linguistic explanation. AI Memo #536, MIT.

Bever, T. G. (1970). The cognitive basis of linguistic structures. In J. R. Hayes, ed. *Cognition and the development of language.* New York: Wiley.

Bever, T. G. (1982). Some implications of the nonspecific bases of language. In E. Wanner and L. Gleitman, eds., *Language acquisition: The state of the art*. New York: Cambridge University Press.

Blumstein, S. (1972). *A phonological investigation of aphasic speech*. The Hague: Mouton.

Blumstein, S., H. Goodglass, S. Statlender, and C. Biber (1983). Comprehension strategies determining reference in aphasia: A study in reflexivization. *Brain and Language* 18, 115–127.

Borer, H. (1979). Passive. Ms., MIT.

Borer, H. (1984). *Parametric syntax*. Dordrecht: Foris.

Borer, H., and Y. Grodzinsky (1986). Syntactic cliticization and lexical cliticization: The case of Hebrew dative clitics. In H. Borer, ed., *Syntax and semantics* 19. San Francisco: Academic Press.

Borer, H., and K. Wexler (1986). The maturation of syntax. In T. Roeper and E. Williams, eds., *Parameter setting and linguistic theory*. Dordrecht: Reidel.

Bouchard, D. (1984). *On the content of empty categories*. Dordrecht: Foris.

Bradley, D. C. (1978). *Computational distinctions of vocabulary type*. Doctoral dissertation, MIT.

Bradley, D. C., M. F. Garrett, and E. B. Zurif (1980). Syntactic deficits in Broca's aphasia. In D. Caplan, ed., *Biological studies of mental processes*. Cambridge, MA: MIT Press.

Bresnan, J. (1978). A realistic transformational grammar. In J. Bresnan, M. Halle, and G. A. Miller, eds., *Linguistic theory and psychological reality*. Cambridge, MA: MIT Press.

Bresnan, J. (1982a). The passive in lexical theory. In Bresnan 1982b.

Bresnan, J., ed. (1982b). *The mental representation of grammatical relations*. Cambridge, MA: MIT Press.

Brown, R., and C. Hanlon (1970). Derivational complexity and order of acquisition in child speech. In J. R. Hayes, ed., *Cognition and the development of language*. New York: Wiley.

Bruner, J. (1973). On perceptual readiness. In J. Anglin, ed., *Beyond the information given*. New York: Norton.

Caplan, D. (1985). Syntactic and semantic structures in agrammatism. In M.-L. Kean, ed., *Agrammatism*. New York: Academic Press.

Caplan, D., and C. Futter (1986). Assignment of thematic roles by an agrammatic aphasic patient. *Brain and Language* 27, 117–135.

Caramazza, A. (1984). The logic of neuropsychological research and the problem of patient classification in aphasia. *Brain and Language* 21, 9–20.

Caramazza, A., and R. S. Berndt (1985). A multi-component deficit view of agrammatic Broca's aphasia. In M.-L. Kean, ed., *Agrammatism*. New York: Academic Press.

Caramazza A., and M. McCloskey (1985). Dissociation of calculation processes. In G. Deloche and X. Seron, eds., *Mathematical disabilities: Cognitive neuropsychological perspective*. Hillsdale, NJ: L. Erlbaum Associates.

Caramazza, A., G. Miceli, and G. Villa (1986). The role of the (output) phonological buffer in reading, writing and repetition. *Cognitive Neuropsychology* 3, 37–76.

Caramazza, A., and E. B. Zurif (1976). Dissociation of algorithmic and heuristic processes in sentence comprehension: Evidence from aphasia. *Brain and Language* 3, 572–582.

Caramazza, A., and E. B. Zurif, eds. (1978a). *Language acquisition and language breakdown*. Baltimore, MD: The Johns Hopkins University Press.

Caramazza, A., and E. B. Zurif (1978b). Comprehension of complex sentences in children and aphasics: A test of the Regression Hypothesis. In Caramazza and Zurif 1978a.

Chomsky, N. (1955/1975). *The logical structure of linguistic theory*. New York: Plenum Press.

Chomsky, N. (1957). *Syntactic structures*. The Hague: Mouton.

Chomsky, N. (1965). *Aspects of the theory of syntax*. Cambridge, MA: MIT Press.

Chomsky, N. (1970). Remarks on nominalization. In R. Jacobs and P. Rosenbaum, eds., *Readings in generative grammar*. Waltham, MA: Ginn.

Chomsky, N. (1977). On wh-movement. In P. Culicover, T. Wasow, and A. Akmajian, eds., *Formal syntax*. New York: Academic Press.

Chomsky, N. (1980). *Rules and representations*. New York: Columbia University Press.

Chomsky, N. (1981). *Lectures on government and binding*. Dordrecht: Foris.

Chomsky, N. (1986a). *Knowledge of language: Its nature, origin, and use*. New York: Praeger.

Chomsky, N. (1986b). *Barriers*. Cambridge, MA: MIT Press.

Chomsky, N. (1988). *Language and problems of knowledge*. Cambridge, MA: MIT Press.

Chomsky, N., and M. Halle (1968). *The sound pattern of English*. New York: Harper and Row.

Clements, G. N., J. McCloskey, J. Maling, and A. Zaenen (1983). String-vacuous rule application. *Linguistic Inquiry* 14, 1–17.

Coltheart, M. (1981). Disorders of reading and their implication for models of normal reading. *Visible Language* 15, 245–285.

Coltheart, M., K. Patterson, and J. C. Marshall, eds. (1980). *Deep dyslexia*. Henley-on-Thames: Routledge and Kegan Paul.

Crain, S., and J. D. Fodor (1985). How can grammars help parsers? In D. Dowty, L. Karttunen, and A. Zwicky, eds., *Natural language processing: Psycholinguistic, computational and theoretical perspectives*. Cambridge: Cambridge University Press.

Crain, S., and C. McKee (1986). Acquisition of structural restrictions on anaphora. *In Proceedings of the Sixteenth Annual Meeting, NELS*. GLSA, University of Massachusetts, Amherst.

Crain, S., and D. Shankweiler (1985). Comprehension of relative clauses and reflexive pronouns by agrammatic aphasics. Paper presented at the Academy of Aphasia, Pittsburgh.

Culicover, P. (1985). Learnability explanations and processing explanations. *Natural Language and Linguistic Theory* 2, 77–104.

Dell, F. (1981). On the learnability of optional phonological rules. *Linguistic Inquiry* 12, 31–37.

Engdahl, E. (1980). Parasitic gaps. *Linguistics and Philosophy* 6, 5–34.

Etcoff, N. (1984). The neuropsychology of emotional expression. Occasional Paper 31, Center for Cognitive Science, MIT.

Fabb, N. (1984). Syntactic affixation. Doctoral dissertation, MIT.

Farah, M. (1985). The neurological basis of visual imagery: A componential analysis. *Cognition* 18, 245–272.

Fodor, J. A. (1975). *The language of thought*. Cambridge, MA: Harvard University Press.

Fodor, J. A. (1981). *Representations*. Cambridge, MA: MIT Press.

Fodor, J. A. (1983). *The modularity of mind*. Cambridge, MA: MIT Press.

Fodor, J. A. (1985). The role of error in causal theories of content. Ms., MIT.

Fodor, J. A., T. G. Bever, and M. F. Garrett (1974). *The psychology of language*. New York: McGraw-Hill.

Fodor, J. A., and M. F. Garrett (1966). Some reflections on competence and performance. In J. Lyons and R. J. Wales, eds., *Psycholinguistic papers. Proceedings of the Edinburgh Conference*. Edinburgh: Edinburgh University Press.

Fodor, J. D. (1985). Learnability and parsability: A reply to Culicover. *Natural Language and Linguistic Theory* 2, 105–150.

Forster, K. I. (1979). Levels of processing and the structure of the language processor. In W. E. Cooper and E. C. T. Walker, eds., *Sentence processing: Psycholinguistic studies presented to Merrill Garrett*. Hillsdale, NJ: L. Erlbaum Associates.

Frazier, L. (1978). *On comprehending sentences: Syntactic parsing strategies*. Doctoral dissertation, University of Connecticut. Distributed by Indiana University Linguistics Club, Bloomington.

Frazier, L. (1986). Natural classes in language processing. Ms., Center for Cognitive Science, MIT.

Frazier, L., C. Clifton, and J. Randall (1983). Filling gaps: Decision principles and structure in sentence comprehension. *Cognition* 13, 187–222.

Freedman, S. E., and K. I. Forster (1985). The psychological status of overgenerated sentences. *Cognition* 19, 101–126.

Friederici, A. (1982). Syntactic and semantic processes in aphasic deficits: The availability of prepositions. *Brain and Language* 15, 249–258.

Friederici, A. (1985). Levels of processing and vocabulary types: Evidence from on-line processing in normals and agrammatics. *Cognition* 19, 133–166.

Friederici, A., P. W. Schonle, and M. F. Garrett (1982). Syntactically versus semantically based computations: Processing of prepositions in agrammatism. *Cortex* 18, 525–534.

Fromkin, V., S. Krashen, S. Curtiss, D. Rigler, and M. Rigler (1974). The development of language in Genie: A case of language acquisition beyond the "critical period." *Brain and Language* 1, 81–107.

Gardner, H., G. Denes, and E. B. Zurif (1975). Critical reading at the sentence level in aphasia. *Cortex* 11, 60–72.

Garrett, M. F. (1975). The analysis of sentence production. In G. Bower, ed., *The psychology of learning and motivation*, vol. 9. New York: Academic Press.

Garrett, M. F. (1980). Levels of processing in sentence production. In B. Butterworth, ed., *Language production. Vol. 1: Speech and talk*. London: Academic Press.

Garrett, M. F. (1982). The organization of processing structure for language production: Implications for aphasic speech. In M. A. Arbib and D. Caplan, eds., *Neural models for language processes*. New York: Academic Press.

Gazdar, G. (1981). Unbounded dependencies and coordinate structure. *Linguistic Inquiry* 12, 155–184.

Gazdar, G., E. Klein, G. Pullum, and I. Sag (1985). *Generalized phrase structure grammar*. Cambridge, MA: Harvard University Press.

Geschwind, N. (1965). Disconnexion syndromes in animals and man. *Brain* 88.2, 237–294; 88.3, 585–644.

Geschwind, N. (1979). Specializations of the human brain. *Scientific American*, September.

Geschwind, N. (1983). Biological foundations of language and hemispheric dominance. In M. Studdert-Kennedy, ed., *Psychobiology of language*. Cambridge, MA: MIT Press.

Goldstein, K. (1948). *Language and language disturbances*. New York: Grune and Stratton.

Goodenough, C., E. B. Zurif, and S. Weintraub (1977). Aphasics' attention to grammatical morphemes. *Language and Speech* 20, 11–19.

Goodglass, H. (1962). Redefining the concept of agrammatism in aphasia. In L. Croatto and C. Croatto-Martinolli, eds., *Proceedings of the XIIth International Speech and Voice Therapy Conference*. Padua, Italy.

Goodglass, H. (1968). Studies in the grammar of aphasics. In S. Rosenberg and J. Koplin, eds., *Developments in applied psycholinguistics research*. New York: Macmillan.

Goodglass, H. (1976). Agrammatism. In H. Whitaker and H. A. Whitaker, eds., *Studies in neurolinguistics*, vol. 1. New York: Academic Press.

Goodglass, H. (1978). Acquisition and dissolution of language. In Caramazza and Zurif 1978a.

Goodglass, H., I. G. Fodor, and C. Schulhoff (1967). Prosodic factors in grammar: Evidence from aphasia. *Journal of Speech and Hearing Research* 10, 5–20.

Goodglass, H., and N. Geschwind (1976). Language disorders (Aphasia). In E. C. Carterette and M. P. Friedman, eds., *Handbook of perception. Vol. 7: Speech and language*. New York: Academic Press.

Goodglass, H., and S. Hunt (1958). Grammatical complexity and aphasic speech. *Word* 14, 197–207.

Goodglass, H., and E. Kaplan (1972). *The assessment of aphasia and related disorders*. Philadelphia, PA: Lea and Febiger.

Goodglass, H., and J. Mayer (1958). Agrammatism in aphasia. *Journal of Speech and Hearing Disorders* 23, 99–111.

Goodglass, H., and L. Menn (1985). Is agrammatism a unitary phenomenon? In M.-L. Kean, ed., *Agrammatism*. New York: Academic Press.

Gordon, B., and A. Caramazza (1982). Lexical decisions for open- and closed-class words: Failure to replicate frequency sensitivity. *Brain and Language* 15, 143–160.

Gordon, B., and A. Caramazza (1983). Closed- and open-class lexical access in fluent and agrammatic aphasics. *Brain and Language* 19, 335–345.

Grimshaw, J. (forthcoming). *Argument structure*. Cambridge, MA: MIT Press.

Grodzinsky, Y. (1984a). The syntactic characterization of agrammatism. *Cognition* 16, 99–120.

Grodzinsky, Y. (1984b). Language deficits and linguistic theory. Doctoral dissertation, Brandeis University.

Grodzinsky, Y. (1985). On the interaction between linguistics and neuropsychology: A review of Noam Chomsky, *On the generative enterprise*. *Brain and Language* 26, 185–195.

Grodzinsky, Y. (1986a). Language deficits and the theory of syntax. *Brain and Language* 27, 135–159.

Grodzinsky, Y. (1986b). Cognitive deficits, their proper description and its theoretical relevance. *Brain and Language* 27, 178–191.

Grodzinsky, Y. (1988). Syntactic representations in agrammatism: The case of prepositions. *Language and Speech* 31, 115–134.

Grodzinsky, Y. (1989). Agrammatic comprehension of relative clauses. *Brain and Language* 31, 480–499.

Grodzinsky, Y. Forthcoming. The fallacy of the recent fad in neuropsychology. Submitted.

Grodzinsky, Y., D. Finkelstein, J. Nicol, and E. B. Zurif (1988). Agrammatic comprehension and the thematic structure of verbs. Paper presented at the Academy of Aphasia, Montreal.

Grodzinsky, Y., and K. Johnson (1985). Principles of grammar and their role in parsing. Ms., MIT.

Grodzinsky, Y., and A. Marek (1988). Algorithmic and heuristic processes revisited. *Brain and Language* 33, 216–225.

Grodzinsky, Y., and A. Pierce (1987). Neurolinguistic evidence for syntactic passive. In *Proceedings of the Seventeenth Annual Meeting, NELS*. GLSA, University of Massachusetts, Amherst.

Grodzinsky, Y., K. Wexler, Y.-C. Chien, and S. Marakovitz (1989). The breakdown of binding relations. Paper presented at the Academy of Aphasia, Santa Fe.

Grossman, M., and S. Haberman (1982). Aphasics' selective deficits in appreciating grammatical agreements. *Brain and Language* 16, 109–120.

Gruber, J. (1965). Studies in lexical relations. Doctoral dissertation, MIT.

Hakuta, K. (1981). Grammatical description versus configurational arrangement in language acquisition: The case of relative clauses in Japanese. *Cognition* 9, 197–236.

Hamburger, H., and S. Crain (1984). The acquisition of cognitive compiling. *Cognition* 17, 85–136.

Heilman, K. (1979). Apraxia. In K. Heilman and E. Valenstein, eds., *Clinical neuropsychology*. New York: Oxford University Press.

Higginbotham, J. (1985). On semantics. *Linguistic Inquiry* 16, 547–593.

Howes, D., and N. Geschwind (1964). Quantitative studies in aphasic language. In D. McK. Rioch and E. A. Weinstein, eds., *Disorders of communication*. Baltimore, MD: Williams and Wilkins.

Huang, J. (1982). Logical relations in Chinese and the theory of grammar. Doctoral dissertation, MIT.

Hyams, N. (1986a). *Language acquisition and the theory of parameters*. Dordrecht: Reidel.

Hyams, N. (1986b). Core and periphery in the acquisition of inflection. Paper presented at the Boston University Conference on Language Acquisition, October.

Isserlin, M. (1922). Über Agrammatismus. *Zeitschrift für die gesamte Neurologie und Psychiatrie* 75, 332–416 (English translation in *Cognitive Neuropsychology* 2, 303–345, 1985).

Jackendoff, R. (1972). *Semantic interpretation in generative grammar*. Cambridge, MA: MIT Press.

Jackendoff, R. (1977). *X' syntax: A study of phrase structure*. Cambridge, MA: MIT Press.

Jackendoff, R. (1987). The status of thematic relations in linguistic theory. *Linguistic Inquiry* 18, 369–411.

Jaeggli, O. (1986). Passive. *Linguistic Inquiry* 17, 587–622.

Jakobson, R. (1941/1968). *Child language, aphasia, and phonological universals*. Originally published in German, published in 1968 by Mouton, The Hague.

Jakobson, R. (1964). Towards a linguistic typology of aphasic impairments. In A. V. S. de Reuck and M. O'Connor, eds., *Ciba Foundation symposium on disorders of language*. London: Churchill.

Jakubowicz, C. (1984). On markedness and binding principles. In *Proceedings of the Fourteenth Annual Meeting*, NELS. GLSA, University of Massachusetts, Amherst.

Johnson, K. (1985). The case for movement. Doctoral dissertation, MIT.

Joos, M. (1954). *Readings in linguistics*. New York: American Council of Learned Societies.

Julesz, B. (1971). *Foundations of the cyclopean perception*. Chicago: University of Chicago Press.

Katz, J. J. (1981). *Language and other abstract objects*. Totowa, NJ: Rowman and Littlefield.

Kean, M.-L. (1977). The linguistic interpretation of aphasic syndromes. *Cognition* 5, 9–46.

Kean, M.-L. (1980). Grammatical representations and the description of language processing. In D. Caplan, ed., *Biological studies of mental processes*. Cambridge, MA: MIT Press.

Kimura, D. (1976). The neural basis of language qua gesture. In H. Whitaker and H. A. Whitaker, eds., *Studies in neurolinguistics*, vol. 2. New York: Academic Press.

Kleist, K. (1934). *Gehirnpathologie*. Leipzig: Barth.

Klosek, J. (1979). Two unargued linguistic assumptions in Kean's "phonological" interpretation of agrammatism. *Cognition* 7, 61–68.

Kolk, H., and M. van Grunsven (1985a). On parallelism in agrammatism. In M.-L. Kean, ed., *Agrammatism*. New York: Academic Press.

Kolk, H., and M. van Grunsven (1985b). Agrammatism as a variable phenomenon. *Cognitive Neuropsychology* 2, 347–384.

Kussmaul, A. (1876). *Die Störungen der Sprache*. Leipzig: Vogel.

Lapointe, S. G. (1983). Some issues in the linguistic description of agrammatism. *Cognition* 14, 1–41.

Lapointe, S. G. (1985). A theory of verb form use in agrammatism. *Brain and Language* 24, 100–155.

Lasnik, H., and J. Kupin (1977). A restrictive theory of transformational grammar. *Theoretical Linguistics* 4, 173–196.

Lasnik, H., and J. Uriagereka (1988). *A course in GB syntax*. Cambridge, MA: MIT Press.

Lenneberg, E. H. (1967). *Biological foundations of language*. New York: Wiley.

Levin, B., and M. Rappaport (1986). The formation of adjectival passives. *Linguistic Inquiry* 17, 623–662.

Lichtheim, K. (1885). On aphasia. *Brain* 7, 433–484.

Lightfoot, D. (1983). *The language lottery: Toward a biology of grammars*. Cambridge, MA: MIT Press.

Linebarger, M. C., M. Schwartz, and E. Saffran (1983). Sensitivity to grammatical structure in so-called agrammatic aphasics. *Cognition* 13, 361–393.

Lukatela, K., S. Crain, and D. Shankweiler (1988). Sensitivity to closed-class items in Serbo-Croat agrammatics. *Brain and Language* 13, 1–15.

Luria, A. R. (1970). *Traumatic aphasia*. The Hague: Mouton.

Lust, B., ed. (1986). *Studies in the acquisition of anaphora*, vol. 1. Dordrecht: Reidel.

McCarthy, J. (1981). A prosodic theory of nonconcatenative morphology. *Linguistic Inquiry* 12, 373–418.

Manzini, M. R., and K. Wexler (1987). Parameters, binding theory and learnability. *Linguistic Inquiry* 18, 413–444.

Marr, D. (1982). *Vision*. San Francisco: W. H. Freeman.

Marr, D., and T. Poggio (1977). From understanding computation to understanding neural circuitry. *Neurosciences Research Program Bulletin* 15. Cambridge, MA: MIT Press.

Marshall, J. C. (1982). Biological constraints on orthographic representation. *Philosophical Transactions of the Royal Society of London* B298, 165–172.

Marshall, J. C. (1985). Foreword. In M. Paradis, H. Hagiwara, and N. Hildebrandt, eds., *Neurolinguistic aspects of the Japanese writing system.* New York: Academic Press.

Marshall, J. C. (1986). The description and interpretation of aphasic language disorder. *Neuropsychologia* 24, 5–24

Marslen-Wilson, W., and L. K. Tyler (1980). The temporal structure of spoken language understanding. *Cognition* 8, 1–71.

May, R. (1977). The grammar of quantification. Doctoral dissertation, MIT.

May, R. (1985). *Logical form: Its structure and derivation.* Cambridge, MA: MIT Press.

Miceli, G., A. Mazzucchi, L. Menn, and H. Goodglass (1983). Contrasting cases of English and Italian agrammatic aphasics. *Brain and Language* 19, 65–97.

Miller, G. A., and N. Chomsky (1963). Finitary models of language users. In R. D. Luce, R. R. Bush, and E. Galanter, eds., *Handbook of mathematical psychology*, vol. 2. New York: Wiley.

Miller, J. L. (1986). Mandatory processing in speech perception: A case study. In J. Garfield, ed., *Modularity in knowledge representation and natural language understanding.* Cambridge, MA: MIT Press.

Mohr, J. P. (1976). Broca's area and Broca's aphasia. In H. Whitaker and H. A. Whitaker, eds., *Studies in neurolinguistics*, vol. 1. New York: Academic Press.

Morton, J. (1982). Brain-based and non-brain-based models of language. In D. Caplan, A. R. Lecours, and A. Smith, eds., *Biological perspectives on language.* Cambridge, MA: MIT Press.

Ojemann, G. (1983). Brain organization from the perspective of electrical stimulation mapping. *Behavioral and Brain Sciences* 6, 189–206.

Osgood, C., and T. A. Sebeok (1954). *Psycholinguistics: A survey of theory and research problems.* Indiana University Publications in Anthropology and Linguistics, Memoir #10.

Panse, F., and T. Shimoyama (1955). Zur Auswirkung aphasischer Störungen im Japanischen. *Archive für Psychiatrie und Zeitschrift für Neurologie* 193, 131–138. (English translation in H. Goodglass and S. Blumstein, eds., 1973, Psycholinguistics and aphasia. Baltimore, MD: The Johns Hopkins University Press.)

Parisi, D., and L. Pizzamiglio (1970). Syntactic comprehension in aphasia. *Cortex* 6, 204–215.

Patterson, K. E. (1981). Neuropsychological approaches to the study of reading. *British Journal of Psychology* 72, 151–174.

Pesetsky, D. (1982). Paths and categories. Doctoral dissertation, MIT.

Pesetsky, D. (1987). Binding problems with experiencer verbs. *Linguistic Inquiry* 18, 126–140.

Peuser, G. (1978) *Aphasie.* Patholinguistica III. Tübingen: W. Fink Verlag.

Pick, A. (1913) *Aphasia.* Trans. Jason Brown. IL: Charles C. Thomas.

Pinker, S. (1982). A theory of the acquisition of lexical interpretive grammars. In Bresnan 1982a.

Pinker, S. (1984). *Language learnability and language development*. Cambridge, MA: Harvard University Press.

Poizner, H., U. Bellugi, and E. Klima (1986). Dissociation between gestural language and gestural programming. Paper presented at the Academy of Aphasia, Nashville.

Reinhart, T. (1983). *Anaphora and semantic interpretation*. London: Croom Helm.

Reinhart, T. (1986). Core and periphery in the grammar of anaphora. In B. Lust, ed., *The acquisition of anaphora*, vol. 1. Dordrecht: Reidel.

Ribot, T. A. (1883). *Les maladies de la mémoire*. Paris: Libraire Germain Baillière.

Riemsdijk, H. van, and E. Williams (1986). *Introduction to the theory of grammar*. Cambridge, MA: MIT Press.

Rizzi, L. (1982). *Issues in Italian syntax*. Dordrecht: Foris.

Rizzi, L. (1985). Two notes on the linguistic interpretation of aphasia. In M.-L. Kean, ed., *Agrammatism*. New York: Academic Press.

Ross, J. R. (1967). Constraints on variables in syntax. Doctoral dissertation, MIT.

Rumelhart, D. E., and J. L. McClelland (1986). On learning the past tense of English verbs. In J. L. McClelland, D. E. Rumelhart, and the PDP Research Group, *Parallel distributed processing: Explorations in the microstructure of cognition*. Vol. 2: *Psychological and biological models*. Cambridge, MA: MIT Press.

Saffran, E., R. S. Berndt, and M. Schwartz (1986). A system for quantifying sentence production deficits in aphasia. Paper presented at the Academy of Aphasia, Nashville.

Saffran, E., M. Schwartz, and O. Marin (1980). The word-order problem in agrammatism: II. Production. *Brain and Language* 10, 263–280.

Schank, R. (1973). Conceptual dependency: A theory of natural language understanding. *Cognitive Psychology* 3, 552–631.

Schuell, H. (1965). *Differential diagnosis of aphasia with the Minnesota Test*. Minneapolis, MN: University of Minnesota Press.

Schwartz, M., M. Linebarger, E. Saffran, and D. Pate (1987). Syntactic transparency and sentence interpretation in aphasia. *Language and Cognitive Processes* 2, 85–113.

Schwartz, M., E. Saffran, and O. Marin (1980). The word-order problem in agrammatism: I. Comprehension. *Brain and Language* 10, 249–262.

Segui, J., J. Mehler, U. Frauenfelder, and J. Morton (1982). The word frequency effect and lexical access. *Neuropsychologia* 20, 615–628.

Sells, P. (1986). *Lectures on Contemporary Syntactic Theories*. Stanford: CSLI.

Shapiro, L., E. B. Zurif, S. Carey, and M. Grossman (1986). Linguistic form-class judgments in agrammatism. Paper presented at the Academy of Aphasia, Nashville.

Simon, H. (1969). *The sciences of the artificial*. Cambridge, MA: MIT Press.

Slobin, D., and T. G. Bever (1982). Children use canonical sentence schemas: A crosslinguistic study of word order and case inflections. *Cognition* 12, 229–265.

Solan, L. (1983). *Pronominal reference: Child language and the theory of grammar.* Dordrecht: Reidel.

Speas, M. (1986). Adjunctions and projections in syntax. Doctoral dissertation, MIT.

Sproat, R. (1986). Competence, performance and agrammatism: A reply to Grodzinsky. *Brain and Language* 17, 160–167.

Stowell, T. (1981). Origins of phrase structure. Doctoral dissertation, MIT.

Swinney, D. (1979). Lexical access during sentence comprehension: (Re)consideration of context effects. *Journal of Verbal Learning and Verbal Behavior* 18, 645–660.

Swinney, D., E. B. Zurif, B. Rosenberg, and J. Nicol (1985). Modularity and information access in the lexicon: Evidence from aphasia. Paper presented at the Academy of Aphasia, Los Angeles.

Taraldsen, T. (1979). On the NIC, vacuous quantification and the that-trace filter. Bloomington, IN: Indiana University Linguistics Club.

Tissot, R. G., G. Mounin, and F. Lhermitte (1973). *L'Agrammatisme.* Brussels: Dessart.

Travis, L. (1984). Parameters and word order variation. Doctoral dissertation, MIT.

Trubetzkoy, N. (1939). *Principles of phonology.* Travaux du cercle linguistique de Prague, VII

Tsvetkova, L. S., and Ah. M. Glozman (1978). *Agrammatizm pri afazii.* Moscow: University of Moscow Press.

Wada, J., and T. Rasmussen (1960). Intracarotid injection of Sodium Amytal for the lateralization of cerebral speech dominance. *Journal of Neurosurgery* 17, 266–282

Warrington, E., and A. Taylor (1973). The contribution of the right parietal lobe to object recognition. *Cortex* 9, 152–164.

Wasow, T. (1977). Transformations and the lexicon. In P. Culicover, T. Wasow, and A. Akmajian, eds., *Formal syntax.* New York: Academic Press.

Wepman, J. M., and L. V. Jones (1964). Five aphasias: A commentary on aphasia as a regressive linguistic phenomenon. In D. McK. Rioch and E. A. Weinstein, eds., *Disorders of communication.* Baltimore, MD: Williams and Wilkins.

Wernicke, K. (1874). *Die aphasische Symptomenkompleks.* Breslau.

Wexler, K., and Y.-C. Chien (1985). The development of lexical anaphors and pronouns. In *Papers and reports on child language development,* 24. Stanford, CA: Stanford University Press.

Wexler, K., and Y.-C. Chien (1988). The acquisition of binding principles. Paper presented at GLOW, Budapest.

Wexler, K., and P. Culicover (1980). *Formal principles of language acquisition.* Cambridge, MA: MIT Press.

Williams, E. (1980). Passive. Ms., University of Massachusetts, Amherst.

Wulfeck, B. (1984). Grammaticality judgment and sentence comprehension in agrammatic aphasia. Paper presented at BABBLE, Niagara Falls, Canada.

Yin, R. K. (1970). Face recognition by brain-injured patients: A dissociable ability. *Neuropsychologia* 8, 395–402.

Zaidel, E., and A. Schweiger (1983). On lexical semantic organization in the brain. In H. Seiler and G. Brettschneider, eds., *Language invariants and mental operations*. Tübingen: Gunter Narr Verlag.

Zurif, E. B., and A. Caramazza (1976). Linguistic structures in aphasia: Studies in syntax and semantics. In H. Whitaker and H. A. Whitaker, eds., *Studies in neurolinguistics*, vol. 2. New York: Academic Press.

Zurif, E. B., A. Caramazza, and R. Meyerson (1972). Grammatical judgments of agrammatic aphasics. *Neuropsychologia* 10, 405–417.

Zurif, E. B., A. Caramazza, R. Meyerson, and J. Galvin (1974). Semantic feature representations in normal and aphasic language. *Brain and Language* 1, 167–187.

Zurif, E. B., H. Gardner, and H. H. Brownell (1989). The case against the case against agrammatism. *Brain and Cognition* 10, 237–255.

Zurif, E. B., and Y. Grodzinsky (1983). Sensitivity to grammatical structure in agrammatism: A reply to Linebarger et al. *Cognition* 15, 207–213.

Zurif, E. B., D. Swinney, and M. F. Garrett (in press). Lexical processing and sentence comprehension in aphasia. In A. Caramazza, ed., *Cognitive neuropsychology and neurolinguistics: Advances in models of cognitive function and impairment*. Hillsdale, NJ: L. Erlbaum Associates.

Name Index

Subject Index

Access routes. *See* Lexicon

Acquisition, 36, 110, 121, 125–127, 143–164, 172n.

Active sentence, 24, 69, 78, 82, 89–90, 92, 99, 119

Agent (theta–role), 31–32, 68, 78, 81–85, 87, 91–92, 115, 121–122, 137–139, 170n.

Agnosia, 3

Agrammatism, 2, 17–18, 22, 37, 39, 77, 136–137, 169n.

  active sentences in, 119–120

  binding in, 125–127, 163

  cleft sentences in, 68, 120

  clinical features of, 17, 38–39, 59

  embedding in, 41–42

  hemiplegia in, 17, 38

  inflection in, 39, 49–50, 56–59

  lexical access in, 42

  morphology and, 49, 52, 60, 118–120

  nonfluency in, 38–39

  passive in, 68–69, 78–80, 118–120, 138

  phonology and, 46–48, 50–53, 57, 147–148

  plural morphemes in, 47

  possessive -s in, 47, 169n.

  prepositions in, 60–61

  relative clauses in, 66, 79, 120

  repetition in, 38

Agreement, 36, 53, 55–56, 58, 149, 164

Alexia, 3, 17

Anaphora (*see also* Coreference, Binding), 35–36, 102–103, 121–125, 153, 155, 160–162

Animacy, 88, 91

Anomic aphasia, 78

Aphasia, 2, 8, 19, 34, 109, 112–114, 120–127, 135, 143–146, 157–158, 163

Aphasic grammar, 54, 56, 147–148, 156–163

Apraxia, 3, 167n.

Arabic, 6

Argument position, 30, 33, 35–36, 87, 93–94

Argument structure, 27-28, 31–34, 42

Behaviorism, 6–7, 131

Bijection Principle, 122

Binding Conditions (*see also* Variable), 25, 35–36, 103, 114, 121–126, 153–156, 160–163

Biological feasibility, 110–112, 129

Brain-behavior relations, 3, 5, 9, 21

Brain damage, 1, 4, 19, 112–113, 144

Broca's aphasia, 2, 10, 39, 43–44, 47–48, 53, 63, 167n. 168n.

  area 37, 168n.

By-phrase, 84, 87, 92, 95, 98, 103

Case studies, 75–77

Case, theory, 25, 34–35, 80, 99, 114–115

C-command, 35, 122–123, 153

Central nervous system, 3, 164

Cerebral localization, 4

Chain (syntactic), 30, 33

Cleft sentence, 68, 79, 82–83, 117, 120

Clitic, 48, 50–51

Closed-class, 12, 39, 43–45, 48, 59, 64, 120

Cognitive impenetrability 133–137

Coindexing. *See* Indexing

Complement, 26–29, 120

Comprehension task, 118–119, 125–127, 163

Computational system, 14

Condition on Extraction Domains, 99

Conduction aphasia, 78

Connectionism, 8–11, 16, 86

Connectionism (PDP), 132